ACCESS Health Press

Destiny's Child No Longer

Rewriting Genetic Fate

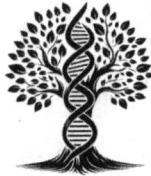

William A. Haseltine Ph.D.
And
Kim Hazel MPH

Acknowledgments

We thank the ACCESS Health US team, Koloman Rath, Amara Thomas, Griffin McCombs, and Roberto Patarca, for their support in creating this book.

This work is supported by ACCESS Health International (www.accessh.org).

Dedication

William Haseltine, Ph.D.

To my wife, Maria Eugenia Maury; my children Mara and Alexander; my stepdaughters Karina, Manuela, and Camila; my grandchildren Pedro Agustin, Enrique Mattias, and Carlos Eduardo; and last but not least, our three dogs, Sky, Luna, and Ginger.

To my mentors and friends, you opened the road and were the wind behind me. Thank you for a wonderful life.

∿

Kim Hazel, MPH

To my loving husband, Colin Purcell.
To my perfect complement, Kelsi McCauley.
To the most brilliant woman I have ever met, Teodora Simion.
To my HOSA Family, Eddie Erickson, and David Guffey.

Books by William A. Haseltine

Affordable Excellence: The Singapore Healthcare Story; William A Haseltine (2013)

Improving the Health of Mother and Child: Solutions from India; Priya Anant, Prabal Vikram Singh, Sofi Bergkvist, William A. Haseltine & Anita George (2014)

Modern Aging: A Practical Guide for Developers, Entrepreneurs, and Startups in the Silver Market; Edited by Sofia Widén, Stephanie Treschow, and William A. Haseltine (2015)

Aging with Dignity: Innovation and Challenge is Sweden-The Voice of Care Professionals; Sofia Widen and William A. Haseltine (2017)

Every Second Counts: Saving Two Million Lives. India's Emergency Response System. The EMRI Story; William A Haseltine (2017)

Voices in Dementia Care; Anna Dirksen and William A Haseltine (2018)

Aging Well; Jean Galiana and William A. Haseltine (2019)

World Class. Adversity, Transformation and Success and NYU Langone Health; William A. Haseltine (2019)

A Family Guide to Covid: Questions and Answers for Parents, Grandparents, and Children; William A. Haseltine (2020)

A Covid Back To School Guide: Questions and Answers for Parents and Students; William A. Haseltine (2020)

Covid Commentaries: A Chronicle of a Plague, Volumes I, II, III, IV, V, and VI; William A. Haseltine (2020)

My Lifelong Fight Against Disease: From Polio and AIDS to Covid-19; William A. Haseltine (2020)

Science as a Superpower: My Lifelong Fight Against Disease And The Heroes Who Made It Possible; William A. Haseltine (2021)

Variants!: The Shape-Shifting Challenge of Covid-19 Vaccine Evasion & Reinfection; William A. Haseltine (2021)

Covid Related Post-traumatic Stress Disorder (CV-PTSD): What It Is And What To Do About It; William A. Haseltine (2021)

Natural Immunity And Covid-19: What It Is And How It Can Save Your Life; William A. Haseltine (2022)

Omicron: From Pandemic to Endemic; William A. Haseltine (2022)

Monoclonal Antibodies: The Once and Future Cure for Covid-19; William A. Haseltine and Griffin McCombs (2023)

The Future of Medicine: Healing Yourself: Regenerative Medicine Part One; William A. Haseltine (2023)

Viroids and Virusoids: Nature's Own mRNAs; William A. Haseltine and Koloman Rath (2023)

CAR T: A New Cure for Cancer, Autoimmune and Inherited Disease; William A. Haseltine & Amara Thomas (2023)

Ending Hepatitis C: A Seven-step Plan for a Successful Eradication Program: A Roadmap for Ending Endemic Disease Globally; William A. Haseltine and Kaelyn Varner (2023)

Better Eyesight*: What You and Modern Medicine Can Do to Improve Your Vision; William A. Haseltine and Kim Hazel (2024)*

Fusion! *The Melding of Human and Machine Intelligence; William A. Haseltine and Griffin McCombs (2024)*

Checkpoint Inhibitors*: A Key to Curing Cancer; William A. Haseltine & Amara Thomas (2025)*

Live Longer*: What You Can Do, What Medicine Can Do; William A. Haseltine and Koloman Rath (2025)*

Recent Textbooks

The COVID-19 Textbook*: Science, Medicine and Public Health; William A. Haseltine and Roberto Patarca (2023)*

Molecular Biology of SARS-CoV-2*: Opportunities for Antivirus Drug Development; William A. Haseltine and Roberto Patarca (2024)*

Contents

Prologue 1

Part I: Decoding Our DNA 3

Chapter 1: The Blueprint of Life: Understanding Our Genetic
Foundation 4

Chapter 2: Deciphering the Code 30

Chapter 3: The Fundamentals of Genes
and Gene Regulation 57

Part II: Rewriting Our Genetic Destiny 72

Chapter 4: The Tools That Are Rewriting Life 73

Chapter 5: Triumphs and Tragedies...109

Chapter 6: Pandora's Box: The Promise and Perils of Genetic
Knowledge 127

Part III: The Future of Genetic Medicine...................................150

Chapter 7: Beyond Disease: Enhancing Human Potential.....151

Chapter 8: From Risk to Routine: Genetic Screening...........168

Chapter 9: The Future Is in Our Genes................................202

References 234

Prologue

What if the hand you were dealt at birth didn't have to define your life?

L ife begins with a silent gamble. A single moment, a microscopic shuffle of DNA, decides the blueprint of who we are. The genetic lottery, they call it. Some are born with a jackpot: robust health, sharp intellect, and resilience encoded into their very being. Others inherit an invisible burden, a script that whispers of future illnesses or limitations, written long before their first breath. It's a roll of the dice that has shaped humanity for millennia, binding us to the double helix of fate.

What if fate could be rewritten?

Imagine holding the threads of your DNA in your hands, no longer a passive recipient of nature's whim but an active author of your story. What if we could decode the mysteries hidden in our genes and use that knowledge to reshape our destinies? The era of genetic medicine is not just on the horizon—**it is here**.

CRISPR and other technologies are no longer confined to laboratories; they are tools poised to redefine what it means to be human. From erasing hereditary diseases to enhancing human potential, science is transforming our DNA from a rigid script into a malleable canvas.

For centuries, humanity has been bound by the limits of biology. Chronic illness, inherited conditions, and predispositions have dictated lives like an unyielding prophecy. But now, gene therapies offer something else: *freedom*. Freedom from the chains of genetic determinism. Freedom to imagine a world where health is not a privilege but a universal right.

This book is your guide into this brave new world—a world where we confront the ethics of rewriting life itself, where the promise of knowledge collides with its perils. Together, we will explore how decoding our DNA can empower us to make informed choices about our health and future. We will examine the tools that allow us to edit genes with precision and consider how society might navigate this unprecedented power.

The ink of our genetic destiny is no longer indelible. We stand at the precipice of possibility, where every cell carries not just the weight of inheritance but the promise of transformation.

Will we use this power wisely? Will we create a future where every individual has the chance to thrive, or will we open Pandora's box, unleashing consequences we cannot foresee?

The choice is ours, collectively and individually.

PART I
Decoding Our DNA

CHAPTER 1

The Blueprint of Life: Understanding Our Genetic Foundation

Amy's hands trembled as she stared at the pristine white envelope on her desk, her name printed in stark black letters. The irony of her situation wasn't lost on her. For years, she had been the calm voice of reason, guiding countless patients through the tumultuous waters of genetic testing. Now, faced with her own reckoning, she felt like a swimmer caught in a riptide, struggling against the very current she had helped others navigate.

The fluorescent lights in her office buzzed overhead, a constant reminder of the sterile world she inhabited every day. But today, the familiar setting felt alien, almost hostile. Amy's eyes darted to the family photo on her desk – a bittersweet reminder of why she sat here, paralyzed by indecision.

Five faces smiled back at her from the frame, five women from her maternal line. All vibrant, all loved, all taken too soon by cancer's relentless grip. Three of them – her mother, aunt, and cousin – had been robbed of even their 40th birthdays. The pattern was undeniable, a grim hallmark of Lynch Syndrome that had woven itself into the very fabric of her family tree.

Amy's mind raced, recalling the countless times she had explained the syndrome to her patients. The words came unbidden, a mantra she had often repeated: "It's a condition caused by mutations in genes responsible for DNA repair. When these are faulty, errors accumulate in the DNA, significantly increasing the risk of cancer development."

But now, those clinical words felt hollow, inadequate to describe the weight of generational trauma that pressed down on her shoulders. Each diagnosis in her family had been another domino falling, another thread unraveling from the tapestry of their shared future. The shadow of it loomed over her like a dark specter, its presence felt in every family gathering, every routine check-up, every passing birthday.

Amy sat at her desk and found herself at the crossroads of professional expertise and raw, personal vulnerability. The central dilemma of our age: *When the blueprint of your life lies before you, inked in the language of DNA, do you dare to read it?*

As she grappled with her decision, Amy felt the weight of decades of research pressing down on her. It was a silent testament to the countless scientists who had dedicated their lives to unraveling the mysteries of DNA, paving the way for this very moment. Their collective knowledge whispered to her, urging her to embrace the power of understanding her own genetic code.

As we embark on this journey, we are setting out on an expedition across uncharted terrain. With each step, we'll uncover new landscapes, navigating the peaks and valleys that reveal how our understanding of DNA has not only changed medicine but also redefined what it means to be human. From the earliest glimpses of DNA's structure to the precision of CRISPR gene editing, we'll follow the winding trail that has brought us to the edge of this vast frontier of knowledge.

But make no mistake – this book is far more than a mere chronicle of scientific milestones. It's a profoundly human saga, pulsing with the hopes, fears, and relentless curiosity of those who've dedicated their lives to decoding our genetic mysteries.

~❧

The journey that made understanding our genetic blueprints a tangible reality began over a century ago with the discovery of DNA. This odyssey, marked by moments of brilliance, serendipity, and relentless determination, would forever change our understanding of life.

In the twilight of the 19th century, a Swiss chemist named Friedrich Miescher stood in his laboratory, the air thick with the acrid scent of chemicals and possibility. His steady hands moved with practiced precision as he carefully isolated a strange, viscous substance from the nuclei of white blood cells. As Miescher held the vial up to the flickering gaslight, he couldn't suppress a shiver of excitement.

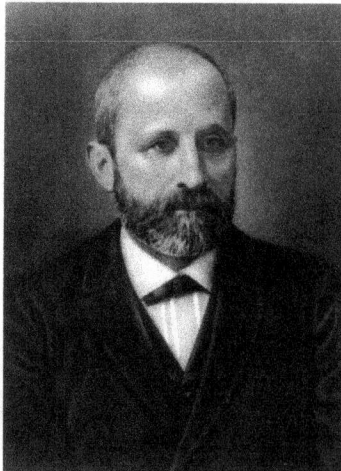

Figure 1. Friedrich Miescher. PBS

The substance, which he dubbed "nuclein," boasted properties that defied conventional wisdom. Little does he know that in his hands, he cradles the very essence of life – *DNA*. With its unusually high phosphorus content and stubborn resistance to protein digestion, nuclein's whispered secrets were yet to be unraveled.

Fast forward to the dawn of the 20th century. In a tranquil monastery garden in Brno, Moravia, a different kind of scientific revolution is quietly unfolding. Gregor Mendel, a bespectacled monk with an uncanny knack for mathematics, kneels in the rich soil, his cassock dusted with pollen. With nothing more than pea plants, meticulous observation, and the patience of a saint, Mendel was poised to change our understanding of heredity and lay the foundation for modern genetics.

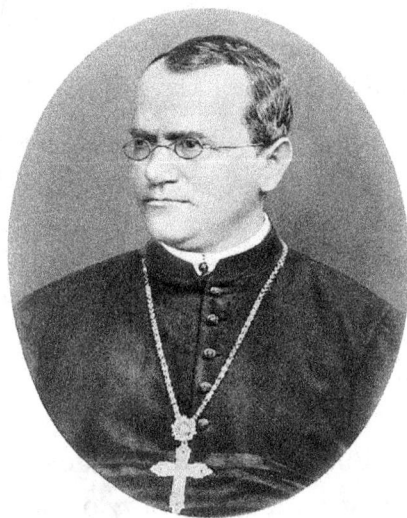

Figure 2. Gregor Mendel. Wellcome Library, London

For seven long years, he nurtured and observed nearly 29,000 pea plants, becoming intimately acquainted with every curl of a leaf and shade of a petal. As his gentle hands brush pollen from one plant to another, playing botanical matchmaker, he's unaware he's about to challenge everything the scientific community believes about heredity. The garden buzzes with bees and the whisper of rustling leaves, nature's own symphony accompanying Mendel's work.

Day after day, season after season, Mendel meticulously records his observations. As the data accumulates, a pattern begins to emerge. Contrary to the prevailing belief that offspring traits were a muddy blend of parental characteristics, Mendel's peas tell a different story. Traits aren't blending like watercolors; they're discrete units, passing from parent to child like perfectly preserved heirlooms.

Mendel discovered that characteristics such as plant height, flower color, and seed shape were controlled by pairs of heritable factors – what we now call genes. He noticed that some traits, like purple flowers, show up easily and often. He called these dominant.

Other traits, like white flowers, can remain hidden and only appear if a plant has the right combination of genes. These are called recessive traits. Little does Mendel know that his work, like a recessive trait, will lie hidden for decades. More than three decades later, his ideas were rediscovered, bursting into bloom and changing the landscape of biology.

In the roaring 1920s, as America swung to jazz rhythms, Dr. Thomas Morgan and his team at Columbia University's "Fly Room" danced to a different tune that would change our understanding of life. The air hummed with the gentle buzz of thousands of fruit flies. Their banana food's sweet, slightly fermented scent permeated the air, mingling with the sharp tang of scientific curiosity.

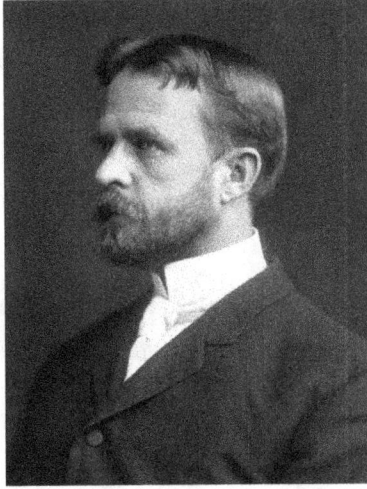

Figure 3. Thomas Morgan. 1891 Johns Hopkins yearbook

Shafts of afternoon sunlight slanted through the windows, catching the translucent wings of thousands of fruit flies as they flitted about their glass homes, creating a shimmering, living kaleidoscope. A single specimen caught Dr. Thomas Morgan's eye. This wasn't just any fruit fly; it was a male with startlingly white eyes—a stark contrast to the typical red-eyed *Drosophila melanogaster.*

As Morgan peered through his magnifying glass, the white-eyed fly seemed to stare back, challenging everything he thought he knew about genes. Its gaze held the key to unlocking mysteries Mendel had only hinted at decades earlier.

With meticulous care, Morgan and his team began breeding this peculiar fly, watching as the white-eye trait appeared and disappeared through generations. Complex and beautiful patterns emerged, like the intricate steps of a cellular dance. These patterns expanded on Mendel's principles, revealing that genes were not just abstract concepts but physical entities with a home on chromosomes.

Morgan pictured genes like beads strung along the length of chromosomes. This model would become known as the chromosome theory of inheritance. Morgan received the 1933 Nobel Prize. Morgan's discoveries brought clarity to the once-murky world of heredity, connecting Mendel's early insights to the rapidly advancing field of genetics.

Yet, even as scientists celebrated these breakthroughs, one crucial question remained unanswered: *What was the actual substance that carried genetic information?*

For years, most believed the answer lay in proteins, given their complexity and variety. But a new chapter was about to unfold. Oswald Avery and his colleagues, Colin MacLeod and Maclyn McCarty, had dared to follow a different trail.

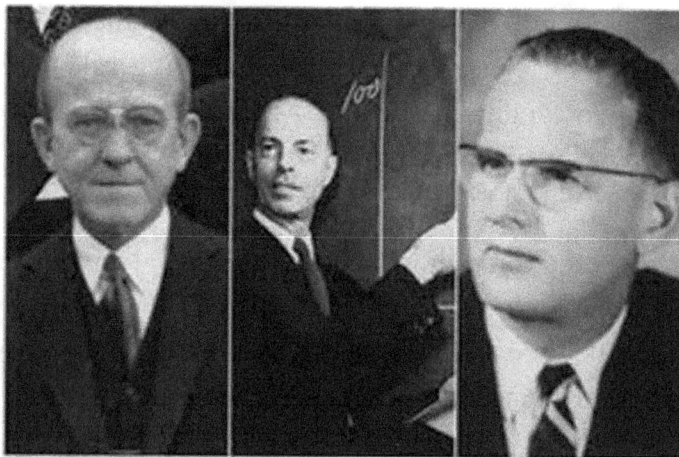

Figure 4. Oswald Avery, Colin Macleod, and Maclyn McCarty. Sutori

The winter of 1944 was bitterly cold, but inside the Rockefeller Institute for Medical Research in New York City, the air simmered with a smoldering anticipation. Their experiments led them to an unexpected conclusion: the transforming principle was not protein but DNA. It had long been dismissed as a simple structural molecule, a minor player in the grand theater of cellular biology. But now, DNA has been revealed as *the architect of life itself.*

The impact of Avery's discovery was seismic. Like a stone cast into a still pond, it sent ripples of excitement and disbelief through the scientific community. In laboratories from New York to London, from Paris to Tokyo, we shifted our gaze to DNA. Microscopes were refocused, hypotheses rewritten, and careers redirected. The race to unravel DNA's secrets had begun in earnest.

As the calendar pages flipped to the early 1950s, in the hallowed halls of Cambridge University's Cavendish Laboratory, two were locked in a frenzied intellectual pursuit. James Watson, bold and young, his wild hair matching his unbridled enthusiasm, and Francis Crick, older and more measured but no less driven, were determined to solve the puzzle that had stumped the scientific world.

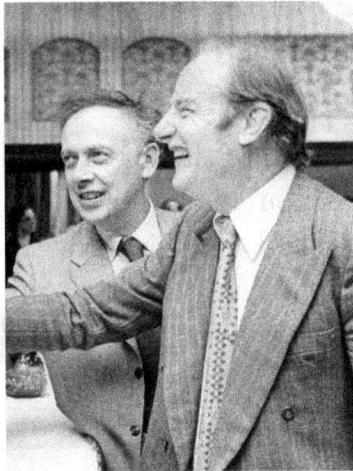

Figure 5. Francis Crick and James D. Watson. Wikimedia Commons

Blackboards erupted with a constellation of equations, their chalk-dusted surfaces a frenzied labyrinth of mathematical hieroglyphs and half-erased theories. Scattered models, intricate skeletal structures of wire, plastic, and gleaming metal, teetered precariously on every available surface, each a fragile monument to their pursuit of understanding.

The air hung heavy with the sharp, acrid tang of coffee mingled with the metallic undertone of electronics and the faint, dusty scent of aging research papers. Voices ricocheted off concrete walls, a symphonic clash of intellects; passionate, argumentative, each scientist's words a verbal jousting match of hypothesis and counter-hypothesis.

Fingers jabbed at diagrams, hands swept dramatically through the air, punctuating complex arguments with the urgency of explorers on the brink of a world-changing discovery. Crumpled paper balls littered the floor, silent witnesses to abandoned theories and midnight epiphanies. Watson and Crick knew that understanding the structure of DNA was more than just an academic exercise—it was the key to unlocking the mystery of life.

Meanwhile, across the bustling streets of London, at King's College, another scientist stood on the precipice of unraveling DNA's enigmatic secrets. Rosalind Franklin, her dark eyes blazing with determination behind fog-smeared laboratory goggles, hunched over her X-ray diffraction apparatus like an alchemist of old. Franklin was a master of her craft, coaxing secrets from crystals that others could only dream of.

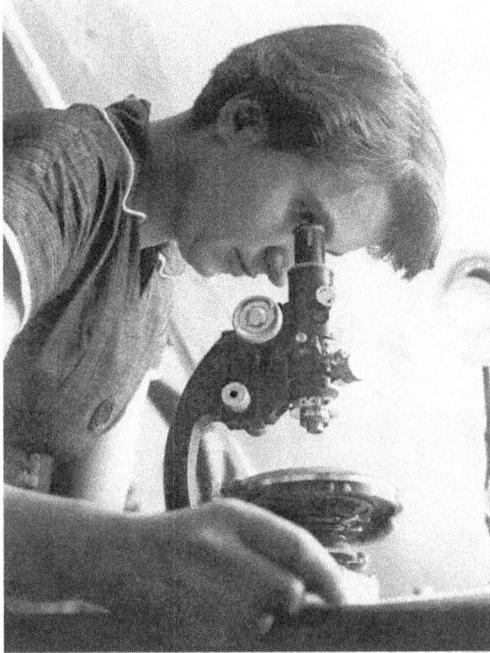

Figure 6. *Rosalind Franklin. MRC Laboratory of Molecular Biology, Wikimedia Commons*

In the crimson-tinged twilight of her darkroom, Franklin's nimble fingers danced through the familiar ritual, coaxing life into her latest X-ray diffraction image. As she gently rocked the developing tray, the ghostly outlines of a pattern began to materialize. Suddenly, the image snapped into focus, and Franklin's breath hitched, caught between a gasp and a whisper.

There, etched in stark monochrome, was a pattern of such exquisite symmetry and elegance. The distinctive "X" shape leapt out at her, a telltale signature of a helical structure. This was Photo 51, an image that would change the course of scientific history.

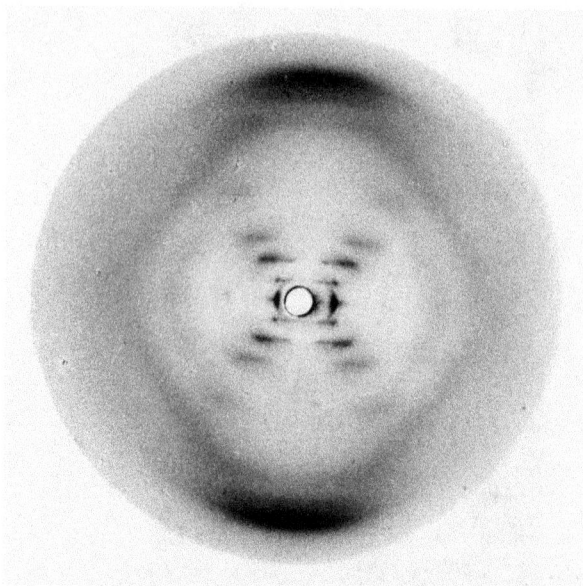

Figure 7. Photo 51. Raymond Gosling at King's College London Archives

The photograph revealed, with unprecedented clarity, the helical structure of DNA. Each dark spot and shadowy arc whispered a cryptic language that Franklin was uniquely equipped to decipher. As she stood transfixed, the dim red light casting an otherworldly glow on her features, Franklin studied the image intently, her mind racing with the implications.

On a frosty February morning in 1953, the air in Cambridge crackled with winter chill. James Watson and Francis Crick stood within the confines of their cluttered office at the Cavendish Laboratory, their eyes ablaze with the feverish gleam of imminent discovery. Hastily scribbled notes adorned every available surface, a frenzied cartography of intellectual exploration. And there lay the X-ray diffraction patterns captured by Rosalind Franklin, snapshots of DNA's hidden architecture.

As the weak winter sun filtered through the frosted windows, Watson's hands moved with a mixture of scientific precision and artistic intuition. The structure, elegant in its simplicity yet profound in its implications, emerged before their eyes. Then, in a moment that would divide scientific history into "before" and "after," everything fell into place.

This wasn't just another hypothesis; the double helix structure explained how DNA could replicate and carry genetic information. The pairs of nitrogenous bases—adenine with thymine and guanine with cytosine—formed the rungs of the ladder, held together by hydrogen bonds. The sugar-phosphate backbones, winding in opposite directions, strengthened and stabilized the structure.

As they rushed to publish their findings, Watson and Crick's excitement was palpable. "We've found the secret of life!" Crick allegedly announced to patrons at the nearby Eagle pub, his words would forever be etched in scientific lore.

Despite this enthusiasm, their paper in *Nature* began with the understated and modest phrase *"We wish to suggest a structure for the salt of deoxyribonucleic acid."* This wasn't just a pretty molecular model; it was the blueprint for all living things.

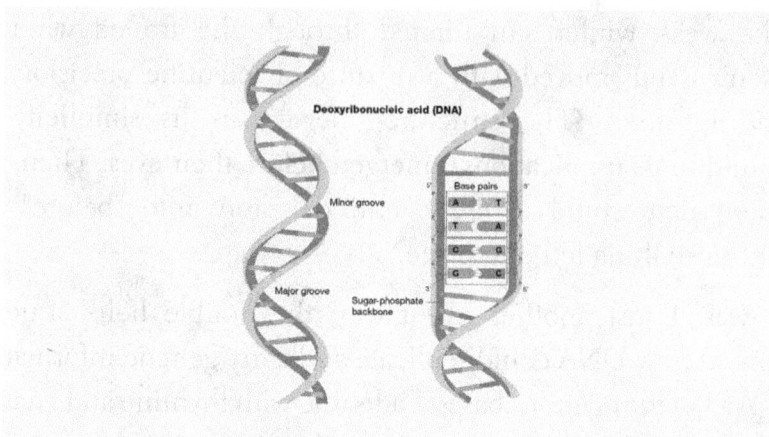

Figure 8. *The physical structure of DNA. National Human Genome Research Institute*

The antiparallel nature of the strands, running in opposite directions like two intertwined spiral staircases, was more than just a structural quirk. It was, as Crick deduced from Franklin's data, the key to understanding how DNA could replicate itself with such fidelity. This insight opened the floodgates to a torrent of new questions and possibilities in the field of molecular biology.

However, perhaps the most profound aspect of their model was the base-pairing rule. The pairing of bases explains how information can be stored, copied, and passed on from one generation to the next. This base-pairing rule means that the sequence of bases on one strand automatically determines the sequence on the complementary strand.

This insight suggested a mechanism for replication. When the two strands are separated, each could serve as a template for a new complementary strand. Moreover, the structure revealed that DNA can contain vast amounts of information.

With four bases that could be arranged in any order along the length of the molecule, DNA had the potential for enormous variability and complexity of the sequence. The structure they had uncovered wasn't just a static molecular scaffold; it was a vibrant, dynamic codex of life, a living library written in the language of four chemical letters.

As Watson and Crick noted, "It follows that in a long molecule, many different permutations are possible, and it, therefore, seems likely that the precise sequence of the bases is the code which carries the genetic information." Like an infinite typewriter ribbon stretching through the nucleus of every living cell, these four characters could be arranged in a dizzying array of combinations.

The implications cascaded through their thoughts. The potential for variability was staggering, almost beyond comprehension. *Trillions upon trillions* of possible arrangements danced before their mind's eye, each one potentially coding for a different trait, a different protein, a different aspect of life, from the curve of a leaf to the firing of a neuron.

This discovery showed that living organisms were not just complex arrangements of matter and energy, but also carriers of information. DNA was revealed to be both a blueprint and a self-replicating machine, capable of storing, copying, and transmitting instructions for building and operating living things. Picture a vast library, where each book contains the instructions for building and operating a living thing.

Every volume in this grand collection contains the intricate blueprints for constructing and operating a living organism, from the simplest bacterium to the most complex mammal. But unlike any earthly library, this one possesses the miraculous ability to duplicate its contents with near-flawless precision, passing its wisdom from one generation to the next in an unbroken chain stretching back to the very dawn of life.

The implications of this discovery rippled through the scientific community like shockwaves. It provided, for the first time, a physical basis for heredity, explaining how traits could be passed from one generation to the next with such remarkable precision. The mystery that had puzzled us since Mendel's time was finally unraveling.

As the initial excitement of discovery settled, a new question emerged that would drive the next phase of genetic research: *How exactly did this molecular marvel copy itself?*

The scientific community found itself at a pivotal juncture in the mid-20th century, grappling with three rival theories to explain this replication: the conservative, dispersive, and semiconservative theories.

In the conservative model, the entire original DNA molecule remains intact, serving as a template to produce a completely new molecule. This leaves one double helix entirely old and the other altogether new after replication. The dispersive model proposed that parental DNA was fragmented during replication, with old and new interspersed in patchwork-like segments along both strands of the daughter molecules. Finally, the semiconservative model suggested that each strand of the original DNA served as a template for a new complementary strand, resulting in daughter molecules composed of one old strand and one newly synthesized strand.

Each offered a distinct vision of how genetic material was copied, but none had yet been proven. In 1958, Matthew Meselson and Franklin Stahl set out to resolve this debate with an experiment.

Using isotopes of nitrogen as molecular markers, they devised an ingenious method to track the behavior of DNA during replication.

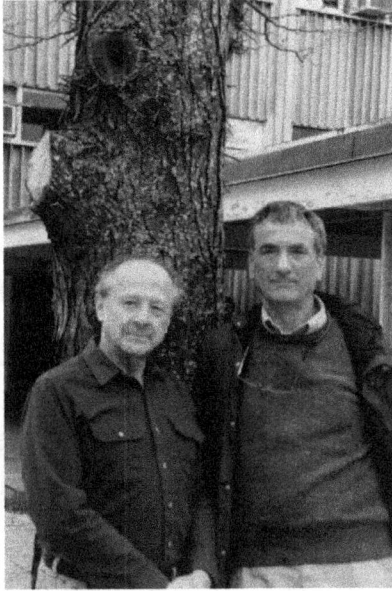

Figure 9. Matt Meselson and Frank Stahl. Courtesy of the Holmes family & ResearchGate

By growing E. coli in a medium enriched with heavy nitrogen and then transferring it to a medium with lighter nitrogen, they labeled the DNA strands in a way that allowed them to distinguish between "old" and "new" strands. With each cycle of replication, they isolated the DNA and subjected it to density-gradient centrifugation. This process separated molecules based on their weight.

After hours of anxious waiting, the centrifuge finally whirred to a stop. Meselson and Stahl leaned in, their eyes fixed on the delicate bands forming in the test tube. The results were unmistakable: after one round of replication, it formed an intermediate band, neither fully heavy nor fully light. After a second round, two distinct bands appeared, one intermediate and one light. The evidence was clear: *DNA replicated semiconservatively.*

At this point, DNA emerged as nature's ultimate multitool. It was at once an architect's blueprint, a master craftsman's instruction manual, and a self-replicating printing press. Its double helix structure, with its complementary base pairs, revealed itself as an ingenious mechanism for both storing and copying the code of life. Each strand served as a template for its partner, ensuring that when the cell divided, two perfect copies of the original blueprint would emerge.

Like a zipper splitting down the middle and being refilled with fresh teeth, each new DNA molecule contained one strand from the original helix and one newly synthesized strand. It was a perfect blend of conservation and innovation, a molecular mechanism that ensured both fidelity and adaptability. This was how life perpetuated itself at the molecular level —a dance of division and replication that had been ongoing since life first appeared on Earth. But the story was far from over.

These past discoveries all led to one nagging question: *How does the information in our genes become the proteins that build and run our bodies?*

In the same transformative year of 1958, molecular biology stood on the brink of yet another revolution. Fresh from his discovery of the double helix, Crick realized that the answer to how our genes came to be was an elegant flow of information. This bold new framework, termed the Central Dogma of Biology, was Crick's attempt to describe the flow of information within living systems.

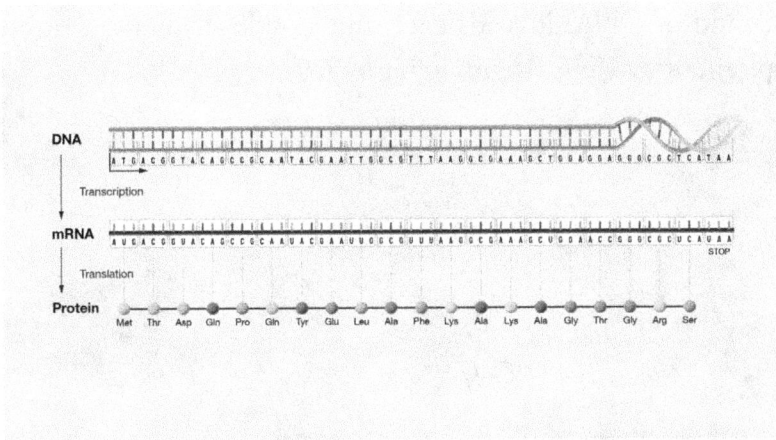

Figure 10. The Central Dogma. National Human Genome Research Institute

He envisioned DNA as more than just a static repository of genetic material—it was the starting point of a one-way cascade of information. Crick proposed that DNA transfers its instructions to RNA. This, in turn, directs the synthesis of proteins. Proteins, however, could not transfer information back to RNA or DNA.

As Crick famously put it, "Once information has passed into protein, it cannot get out again."

At the heart of this process lie two fundamental steps: transcription and translation. In transcription, the cell performs an act of molecular scribing, carefully copying a gene from DNA into a portable format called messenger RNA, mRNA. It's as if a chef were jotting down a treasured recipe from the sacred cookbook of DNA onto a slip of paper. This mRNA is the portable blueprint, ready to leave the nucleus' library and enter the cell's bustling kitchen.

With the precision of a master, an enzyme called RNA polymerase unzips the double helix, separating its intertwined strands to reveal the genetic instructions hidden within. Moving methodically along one strand of DNA, it reads each nucleotide. It then assembles a complementary RNA strand, letter by letter.

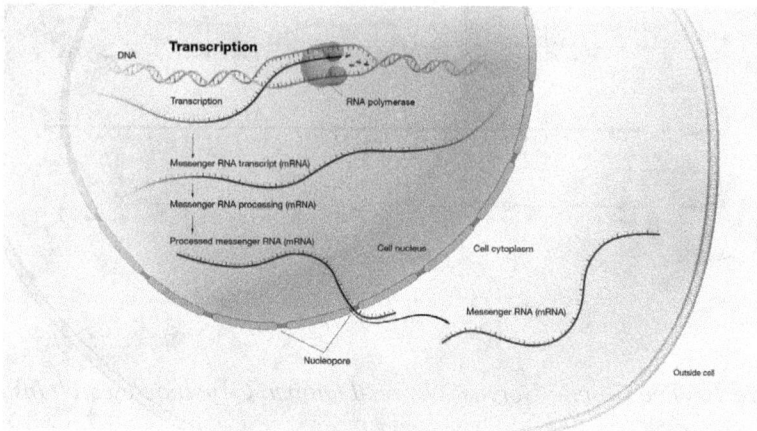

Figure 11. Transcription. National Human Genome Research Institute

This newly minted mRNA is a faithful transcript of the original recipe. It captures the sequence of genetic information. Once complete, this molecular recipe leaves the nucleus and enters the cytoplasm, where it will face its next challenge: translation.

In translation, the mRNA's instructions are "read" by cellular machines called ribosomes. If transcription is akin to jotting down a recipe, translation is like assembling a gourmet dish from scratch. The ribosome acts as a meticulous sous-chef, reading the mRNA's sequence and translating it into the language of amino acids, the building blocks of proteins. These ribosomes are the true artisans of the cellular world, capable of reading the code and translating it into the language of proteins.

Cell nucleus

RNA polymerase

Transcription

Translation

Growing polypeptide chain

tRNA

Peptide moves
to the next tRNA

mRNA

tRNA

tRNA

tRNA

Cell cytoplasm

mRNA

CCAGUGUCAGGAUCACG ... Codons

Ribosome

Outside cell

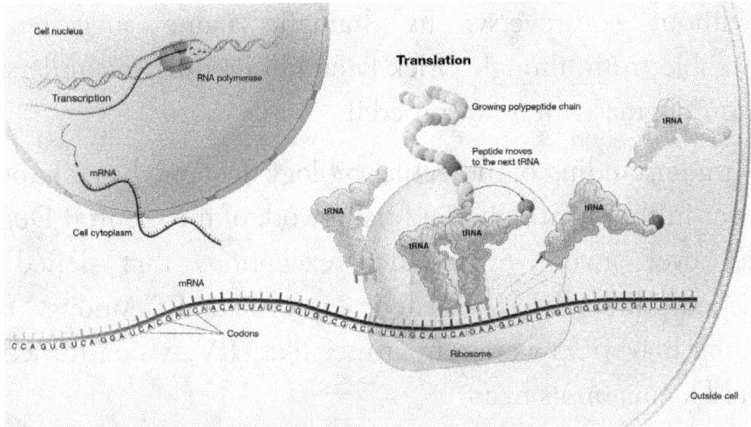

Figure 12. Translation. National Human Genome Research Institute

As the mRNA threads through the ribosome, each set of three nucleotide bases - a codon - is carefully read. Each codon serves as a molecular shorthand for an amino acid, much like culinary symbols that specify ingredients for a dish. Transfer RNA, tRNA, molecules act as couriers in this process. They ferry specific amino acids to the ribosome. Each tRNA carries an anticodon that matches up with its corresponding codon on the mRNA, ensuring that every ingredient is added in precisely the correct order.

With each codon read and each amino acid delivered, the ribosome stitches together a growing chain of amino acids. Slowly but surely, this chain folds into a unique three-dimensional structure, a protein, ready to perform its role in sustaining life. From enzymes that catalyze chemical reactions to structural proteins that give cells their shape, these molecular creations are as diverse as they are essential.

Together, transcription and translation form one of biology's most elegant symphonies: a seamless flow to functional molecules. It is in these steps that DNA's promise is fulfilled—this elegant flow of information, from DNA to RNA to protein. The Central Dogma was not without controversy. Its dramatic name suggested an unshakeable truth, though Crick later admitted he misunderstood the term "dogma" when he coined it.

As our understanding of molecular biology deepened, cracks began to appear in the seemingly rigid framework of the Central Dogma. Nature, ever inventive, revealed exceptions that defied the established direction of genetic information. Among these molecular mavericks were retroviruses like HIV, which turned the Central Dogma on its head.

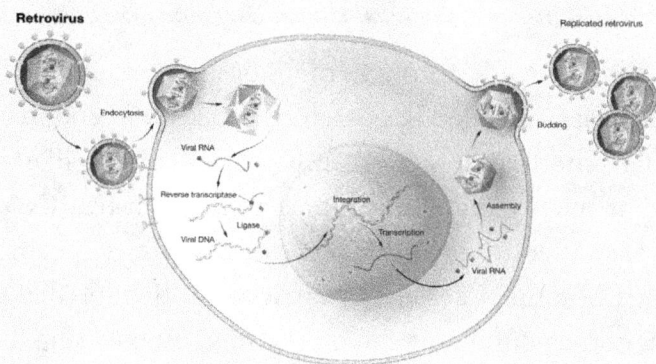

Figure 13. Retroviruses. National Human Genome Research Institute

These retroviruses possess an enzyme called reverse transcriptase, which enables them to reverse the flow of information by converting RNA into DNA—a process aptly named reverse transcription. It's as if they've found a way to recreate the master recipe from a hastily scribbled note. They rewrite the rules to suit their survival strategies.

But nature's surprises didn't end there. The discovery of non-coding RNAs added yet another layer of complexity to our understanding of life's molecular machinery. Once dismissed as mere intermediaries or "junk," these RNA molecules emerged as potent regulators within the cell. They orchestrated intricate processes, from controlling gene expression to maintaining chromosomal stability.

Among these discoveries, RNA interference further complicated the picture, showing that some RNA molecules could silence genes. Picture a sous-chef in the cellular kitchen, deftly covering specific recipes in the genetic cookbook, ensuring they remain unused. RNAi operates through small RNA molecules that guide specialized protein complexes to target messenger RNAs for degradation or translational suppression. This mechanism not only regulates expression but also plays a critical role in defending against viral infections and maintaining genomic integrity.

Together, these discoveries shattered the simplicity of the Central Dogma. They unveil a dynamic molecular world where information flows in unexpected directions and RNA takes on roles far beyond its traditional intermediary function. Yet despite its speculative origins and later discoveries of exceptions, the Central Dogma became the cornerstone of molecular biology.

It provided a unifying framework for understanding how genetic information is stored, expressed, and transmitted. This is a conceptual leap as profound as the discovery of DNA's structure itself. The dogma served as a foundational scaffold for molecular biology, offering a clear pathway to explain the fundamental processes of life. Over time, this principle became the bedrock upon which generations built our modern understanding of expression, heredity, and cellular function.

As the 1960s dawned, the scientific community turned its attention to deciphering the language of life itself: the genetic code. Marshall Nirenberg and Heinrich Matthaei set out to crack the code—*the language of life.* The code, they discovered, was an intricate system of triplet codons; three-letter sequences of nucleotides that encoded specific amino acids. This universal language, spoken by nearly all living organisms, revealed the elegant simplicity underlying life's staggering complexity.

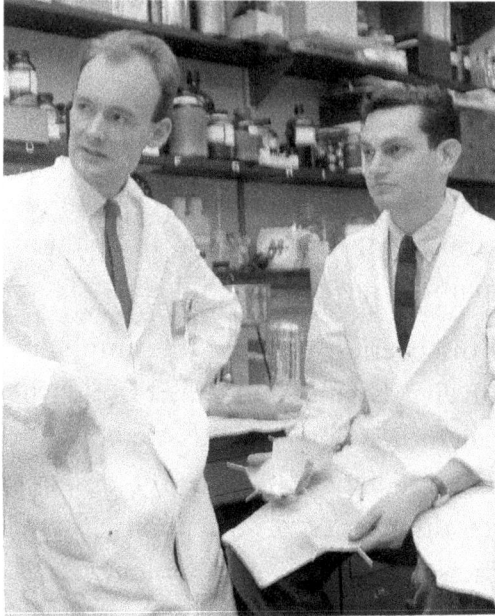

Figure 14. Marshall Nirenberg and Heinrich Matthaei. Norman MacVicar, NIH photographer

It stands as biology's Rosetta Stone, a universal cipher that translates the four-letter alphabet of DNA into the twenty-letter lexicon of proteins, which are made up of amino acids. This code ensures the faithful transmission of genetic information across generations, from the nucleus to the cellular machinery.

In their quest to crack this code, they worked with tireless precision, crafting synthetic RNA molecules and observing which amino acids they summoned into existence. Their laboratory became a crucible of discovery, each experiment an act of molecular translation. It was painstaking work, hours spent coaxing meaning from sequences of nucleotides, but their persistence bore fruit. They deciphered the first "word" of the genetic code, the sequence UUUU. This simple triplet encodes the amino acid phenylalanine, which is essential to life.

With this breakthrough, they had done more than solve a puzzle; they had opened a door to a future where humanity might one day rewrite the very fabric of life. The code, it turned out, was a universal language, a shared heritage that unites all living organisms in existence. The same code that governs human cells also governs those of trees, whales, and microbes.

From the humblest bacterium swimming in a drop of water to the most complex human being pondering their place in the cosmos, every living thing relies on this code to translate genetic instructions into proteins—the molecular architects and laborers that build and sustain life.

The elegance of the genetic code, with its precise translation of DNA into proteins, also revealed its inherent vulnerability. Like a finely tuned symphony, even the slightest disruption could throw the entire composition into disarray. When genes go awry, the consequences can be profound. Mutations or changes in the DNA sequence can disrupt the delicate equilibrium of protein synthesis, leading to diseases that affect an organism's development and function.

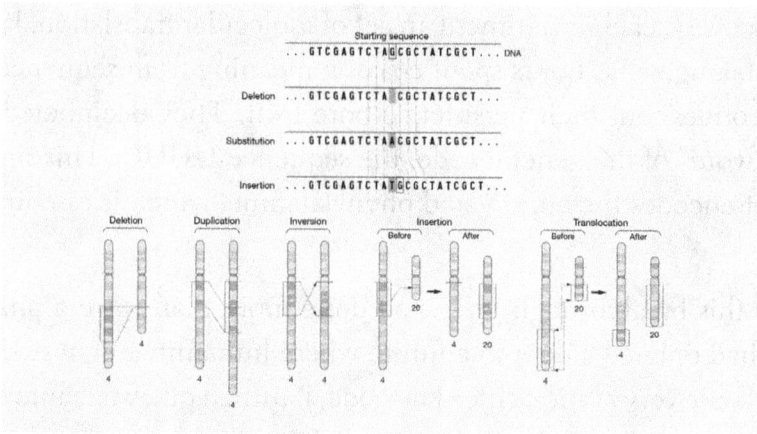

Figure 15. Genetic Mutations. National Human Genome Research Institute

These errors in the code come in many forms, each a molecular glitch with potentially devastating effects. Some are as subtle as a single nucleotide substitution, a solitary typo in the vast manuscript of life's instructions. Others are more catastrophic: large-scale deletions, duplications, or rearrangements of genetic material that can rewrite entire chapters of the genome. Each mutation carries its own story, its own impact on the intricate machinery of life.

Consider sickle cell anemia, one of the most striking examples of how a tiny alteration can have far-reaching consequences. This debilitating condition is marked by misshapen red blood cells that struggle to carry oxygen through the body. Armed with their newfound understanding of the code, we traced this disease back to its source: a single nucleotide mutation in the hemoglobin gene.

Just one letter in a sequence of billions, an adenine swapped for a thymine, caused a single amino acid change in hemoglobin, transforming it into a molecule that clumped together and distorted red blood cells into their characteristic sickle shape. This minuscule error, a molecular whisper in the genome's vast expanse, was enough to wreak havoc on those affected, leading to chronic pain, organ damage, and reduced life expectancy.

For the first time, we could trace the origins of disease to the molecular level, peeling back the layers of mystery that had shrouded conditions like sickle cell anemia for centuries. And so, new questions began to take shape… questions that would define the future of science and humanity itself: *If we could read the book of life, could we also edit it? Rewrite its flawed passages, correcting errors that brought so much pain*

CHAPTER 2

Deciphering the Code

O nce confined to the pages of science fiction, our ability to decipher the genetic code has grown exponentially since Mendel's days with his pea plants. But understanding the code is only the beginning. The true power lies not just in reading the script of life but in rewriting it—*reshaping* our genetic fate with precision and purpose.

As we stand on the precipice of this new era in medicine, the stories of real people remind us of the profound impact these scientific advances can have on individual lives. No longer are we passive spectators to the whims of our genetic inheritance; we are becoming architects of our own biology. The world was on the brink of a seismic transformation, and a quiet revolution was already brewing in laboratories across the globe.

In one such lab at the University of Tennessee, biochemist Lorraine Kraus burned the midnight oil, her eyes fixed on the microscope. Her determination burned as brightly as the fluorescent light above her workstation. The rhythmic hum of centrifuges and the gentle clinking of test tubes formed a symphony of discovery as she worked tirelessly to unravel the mysteries of genetic disorders.

Kraus had a vision: *What if we could go beyond treating symptoms and instead correct genetic disorders at their very source? What if we could introduce healthy DNA into diseased cells, repairing them from within?*

Using a technique known as DNA-mediated gene transfer, Kraus carefully combined bone marrow cells from a patient with sickle cell with healthy donor DNA. The goal was to introduce a functional beta-globin gene into the patient's cells, correcting the defect at its very root. The process was as intricate as it was ambitious, requiring precision at every step.

The process starts with isolating the healthy gene from a donor. Next, the patient's bone marrow cells need to be prepared, stripping them down to their molecular essence to make them receptive to this new genetic instruction. Finally, the healthy DNA is integrated into the patient's chromosomes to see if the modified cells can produce normal hemoglobin. If successful, these modified cells would produce normal hemoglobin, restoring balance to a system thrown into chaos by a single mutation.

Kraus held her breath as she peered through her microscope. Before her eyes, something magical was happening: the patient's cells were producing normal hemoglobin. She had successfully incorporated functional DNA into mammalian cells, altering their makeup at its very core. It was proof that the genetic code could be more than a record of inheritance—it could be rewritten, repaired, and redeemed. Her work laid the foundation for what would become modern gene therapy.

As news of Kraus's discovery spread through the scientific community, it ignited a firestorm of research and speculation. Kraus's work represented a lifeline. It was a promise that our genetic fate might not be set in stone. While it would take decades for gene therapy to transition from the sterile confines of the laboratory to the bustling corridors of clinics, the seeds had been firmly planted.

Using Kraus's work as a basis for further research, a trio at the National Institutes of Health, Theodore Friedmann, Jay Seegmiller, and John Subak-Sharpe, set their sights on an even more formidable challenge: Lesch-Nyhan syndrome. This rare and devastating neurological disorder, first described in 1964, was known to cause severe neurological abnormalities, compulsive self-injurious behavior, and overproduction of uric acid.

Their trial involved the same meticulous process as Kraus's work. With painstaking precision, the team embarked on a trial that mirrored Kraus's process. They first isolated the gene responsible for the enzyme deficiency at the heart of the syndrome, a molecular needle in the vast haystack of the human genome. Next, they prepared the patient's cells, creating a cellular canvas ready to receive the healthy gene.

The results, when they came, were both exhilarating and humbling. A small number of the patient's cells—*about one in a million*, a fraction so minuscule it seemed almost insignificant—showed evidence that the defect had been corrected. It was *a whisper of success*, barely audible above the background noise of cellular processes, yet it echoed with profound implications. This victory was proof that even the most complex genetic disorders could potentially be addressed at their very source.

These efforts, though confined to the controlled environment of the laboratory, marked strides toward the development of gene therapy. They demonstrated that correcting genetic defects at the cellular level was not just a theoretical possibility but a tangible reality. In petri dishes across the world, we were rewriting the rules of genetics, one cell at a time. Each successful gene transfer, no matter how small, was a step towards a future where diseases might be relegated to the annals of history.

As the 1970s dawned, science stood on the threshold of a transformative era. Amid the backdrop of the Apollo moon landings and humanity's first steps beyond Earth, another frontier was quietly being explored here on the ground: *the genetic code.* Gene therapy, still in its infancy, was beginning to take its first tentative steps toward clinical reality.

In 1977, Frederick Sanger, a quiet biochemist at the University of Cambridge, introduced a method that forever altered the trajectory of genetics and medicine. Known as Sanger sequencing, this technique unlocked the ability to read the precise order of nucleotides that compose DNA. For the first time, we could decipher the instructions encoded within the double helix.

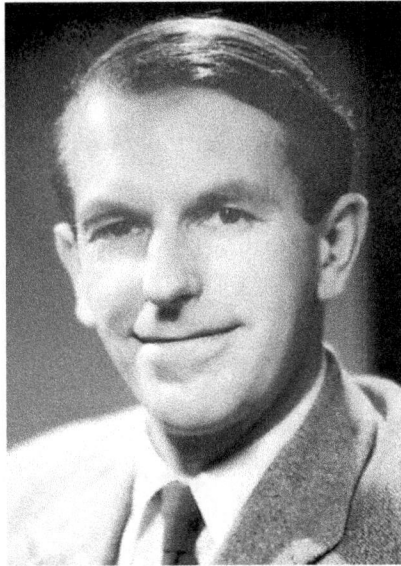

Figure 16. Frederick Sanger. The Nobel Foundation

Before Sanger sequencing, deciphering even short DNA sequences was an arduous and imprecise endeavor. His chain-termination or dideoxy method solved this problem. It used modified nucleotides called dideoxynucleotides, which lack the chemical group necessary for strand elongation.

Sanger devised a way to halt DNA synthesis at specific points. This process generated fragments of varying lengths, each terminating at a particular nucleotide. These fragments were then separated by size, and their terminal bases were identified via radioactive or fluorescent labels. The result was a readable sequence of DNA, a molecular code laid bare with clarity and precision.

Sanger sequencing was not just groundbreaking for its accuracy but also for its practicality. It transformed sequencing from an abstract concept into a tangible reality, enabling the sequencing of entire genes and even small genomes with relative efficiency. Sanger demonstrated his method's power by sequencing a bacteriophage's genome. Specifically, a virus that infects *E. coli.* This achievement marked the first complete genome ever sequenced, a milestone that showcased his technique's potential and set the stage for its widespread adoption.

The impact of Sanger sequencing rippled across biology and medicine. It became the gold standard for over two decades, empowering us to map genes, identify mutations, and unravel the molecular basis of countless diseases. Sanger's work provided a molecular map to pinpoint mutations with precision, guiding efforts to correct defects at their source. His method enabled us to locate errors in the code with unparalleled accuracy—a critical step in developing targeted treatments for genetic disorders.

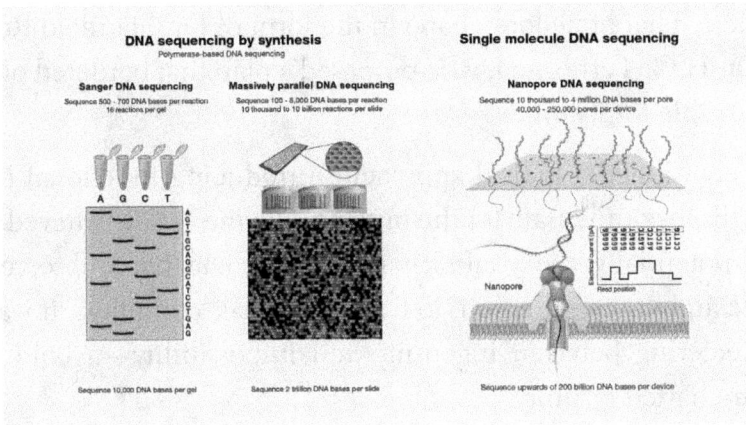

Figure 17. DNA Sequencing. National Human Genome Research Institute

Frederick Sanger's contribution was more than technical; it was foundational. His sequencing method gave us a tool and an entirely new lens through which to view life. By transforming DNA from an enigmatic molecule into a readable script, he opened doors to discoveries that would shape the future of biology and medicine.

~

In 1972, far from the bustling laboratories of Cambridge where Sanger's innovations were taking shape, two young sisters, Greta and Ingrid, faced a future overshadowed by a rare and relentless genetic disorder: hyperargininemia. For Greta and Ingrid, the disorder was relentless. The condition prevents the production of an enzyme called arginase. For Greta and Ingrid, it meant severe neurological problems, brain damage, and epilepsy loomed as inevitable consequences.

Their parents watched helplessly as the disease tightened its grip on their daughters' lives. Yet amidst their heartbreak, they clung to hope: a fragile but persistent belief that science might one day offer salvation. That hope took shape in the form of Dr. Stanfield Rogers and Dr. H.G. Terheggen, who proposed a plan that bordered on the unthinkable for its time.

They envisioned a radical approach: introducing functional DNA into cells to compensate for the missing enzyme. They believed they could potentially use a rabbit virus, which had been observed to induce arginase production, to treat the sisters' condition. It was an idea teetering between ingenuity and impossibility—a bold leap into uncharted territory.

The process they imagined would involve isolating healthy DNA containing the arginase gene and delivering it into Greta and Ingrid's cells in hopes of restoring normal function. The science behind this approach was both clever and risky, as well as mostly rejected by the medical science community at large.

Dr. Stanfield Rogers and his team turned to the Shope papillomavirus, a virus first discovered in the 1930s that caused horn-like warts in rabbits. What set this virus apart wasn't just its peculiar pathology but its surprising ability to induce the production of arginase, the very enzyme Greta and Ingrid's bodies couldn't produce due to their disorder.

The idea was that if the virus could stimulate arginase production in rabbit cells, its genetic machinery could be harnessed to do the same in human cells. Rogers hypothesized that the viral DNA, once introduced into Greta and Ingrid's cells, might integrate into their genomes and act as a biological factory, producing the missing enzyme. It was one of the earliest attempts at what we now call gene therapy: using genetic material to treat disease at its source.

The day of treatment dawned heavy with anticipation and fear, a cocktail of emotions that hung heavy in the air. Greta and Ingrid, sisters bound by love and by the cruel grip of hyperargininemia, received their injections. These were no ordinary injections; they were among the first *"viral vector"* treatments ever attempted, designed to deliver corrected material directly into their cells.

The weeks that followed were an emotional whirlwind. Greta and Ingrid's parents swung between cautious hope and deep worry. Every small sign of improvement sent their spirits soaring; every setback brought them crashing down. The medical team felt the same tension, eagerly scanning lab results and clinical observations for any sign that the treatment was working and correcting the issue.

Then, as if fate had a cruel sense of timing, a third sister was born, also afflicted with hyperargininemia. The family faced an agonizing decision: *should they subject their newborn daughter to the same experimental treatment?*

With hope tempered by the lessons learned from Greta and Ingrid's journey, they chose to proceed. The infant received her own injection of viral vectors, and once again, doctors monitored her progress with unwavering vigilance.

Months passed, and the initial excitement began to wane. Despite their best efforts, neither Greta nor Ingrid nor their younger sister showed any improvement. The treatment failed to stimulate arginase production or alleviate their condition. The disappointment was profound, a heavy weight on the shoulders of both the medical team and the family who had pinned their hopes on this experimental approach. Dr. Rogers and his team did not achieve the breakthrough they hoped for.

Still, amidst the sorrow of unmet expectations, there was a silver lining. Though unsuccessful, this early attempt at gene therapy marked a crucial first step in the journey of genetic intervention.

Greta and Ingrid's story became more than a tale of heartbreak; it became a rallying cry around the world.

It underscored the importance of perseverance in science, the willingness to take risks even when success seems elusive. This early experiment represented a seismic shift in medicine: from passively accepting genetic disorders as fate to proactively seeking ways to rewrite life's blueprint. This shift from passive acceptance to proactive intervention in more modern times is perhaps best illustrated by the case of a young girl whose story would help usher in a new chapter in genetic treatment years later.

~❧

In a sterile hospital room, a four-year-old girl named Ashanthi DeSilva faced a battle that no child should have to fight. Diagnosed with severe combined immunodeficiency, her world was a fragile bubble where every breath carried danger and every touch posed a threat. The hospital room, with its stark white walls and the hum of air filters, became her fortress against an outside world teeming with invisible enemies. The beeping monitors and rhythmic hiss of machinery created a mechanical symphony that underscored the fragility of her existence.

Her parents, donning protective gear just to hold her hand, longed for the day they could embrace their daughter without fear, to feel her skin against theirs without the interference of gloves and masks. The layers of sterile material between them were a cruel metaphor for the barrier that the immunodeficiency had erected between Ashanthi and the world. Each day was a tightrope walk between hope and despair, their hearts breaking with every labored breath their little girl took. They watched helplessly as Ashanthi's condition deteriorated.

Ashanthi's plight didn't go unnoticed. It captured the attention of Dr. W. French Anderson, a geneticist at the National Institutes of Health's National Heart, Lung, and Blood Institute. As he pored over Ashanthi's case files late into the night, the fluorescent lights of his office casting long shadows, an idea began to take shape. The idea was to introduce a healthy gene into Ashanthi's cells to correct the genetic defect at its source. It was a molecular-level intervention to rewrite the faulty code in Ashanthi's DNA.

At the heart of his plan was a retroviral vector, a modified virus designed to act as a molecular Trojan horse. This wasn't just any virus; it was a carefully crafted vehicle designed to smuggle healthy genes past the body's defenses. It would carry a healthy copy of the ADA gene into Ashanthi's cells, integrating it into her DNA.

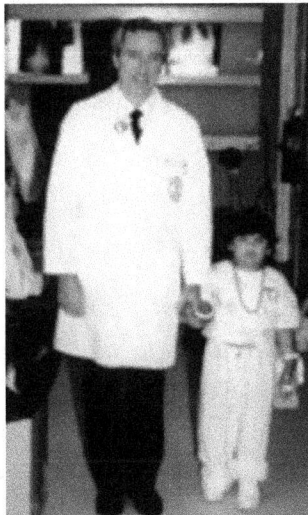

Figure 18. Ashanthi with Dr. W. French Anderson. Original Publication by PBS

On September 14, 1990, Ashanthi DeSilva, with wide, curious eyes, lay on the bed. Her tiny body was dwarfed by the medical equipment surrounding her. Her parents, their faces a mixture of hope and fear, stood by her side, their hands clasped tightly together.

Ashanthi received an infusion of her own white blood cells that had been genetically modified outside her body. The cells, now carrying the gene responsible for producing adenosine deaminase, were reintroduced into her bloodstream. As the infusion began, time seemed to slow to a crawl. The soft beep of monitors and the hushed whispers of the medical team faded into the background.

All eyes were fixed on the thin tube carrying the modified cells into Ashanthi's bloodstream. Each drop that fell was a step into uncharted territory, a bold leap into the realm of genetic medicine. This wasn't just about saving one little girl; it was about opening the door to a future where diseases could be corrected at their source.

Weeks turned into months, and the medical team watched Ashanthi with hawk-like intensity. Every blood test was scrutinized, and every scan was analyzed with painstaking detail. Slowly, almost imperceptibly at first, signs of improvement began to emerge. Ashanthi's immune system, once as fragile as spun glass, showed resilience. Blood tests revealed a gradual increase in her white blood cell count.

Her body was beginning to defend itself for the first time.

The changes weren't just clinical. Ashanthi's parents noticed a new spark in their daughter's eyes, a vitality that had been absent. She laughed more, played longer, and embraced life with a newfound energy. For the first time, they dared to hope for a future where their daughter could live free from the constant threat of infection.

As Ashanthi's strength grew, so did the excitement in the scientific community. Her case was meticulously documented, every improvement celebrated as a milestone not just for her, but for the entire field of gene therapy. Though not a complete cure, Ashanthi still required supplemental enzyme therapy and recurrent treatment. She received 11 infusions across a two-year span. The therapy strengthened her immune system enough for her to experience life beyond hospital walls.

Her case became a focal point of hope and possibility, meticulously documented with every small improvement celebrated as a milestone, not just for her, but for the burgeoning field of gene therapy. She was living proof that the once-fantastical idea of rewriting our genetic code was possible and could be life-changing. As she grew stronger, so did the resolve worldwide to push the boundaries of medicine.

"We basically showed that you could do this, you could do it safely, and you could have a positive impact on patients," Dr. R. Michael Blaese, chief of the Cellular Immunology Section of the NIH's National Cancer Institute, later told GEN. "It wasn't a curative trial, but it was certainly an effective treatment, and I think it did open the door for some very successful trials that have cured patients of a number of diseases."

For families grappling with genetic disorders, Ashanthi's story was like the first glimmer of dawn after an endless night. Support groups buzzed with excited conversations about gene therapy trials, and parents of children with SCID or other conditions began asking their doctors about this treatment. Ashanthi's journey gave them something they had long been denied: hope.

The dawn of gene therapy had arrived. Ashanthi's brave journey had opened a door, one through which countless others would follow. Each step forward brought humanity closer to a world where genetic diseases could be treated or even cured. As the excitement surrounding Ashanthi's success continued to build, another chapter in the story was about to unfold.

~•

Amid the growing momentum of gene therapy's promise, Jesse Gelsinger stood as a symbol of quiet bravery, his optimism unshaken despite the invisible battle raging within his cells. He suffered from ornithine transcarbamylase deficiency, known as OTC, a rare genetic disorder that left his body unable to break down ammonia, a toxic byproduct of protein metabolism. This condition, which affects approximately 1 in every 40,000 newborns, is often fatal within days of birth.

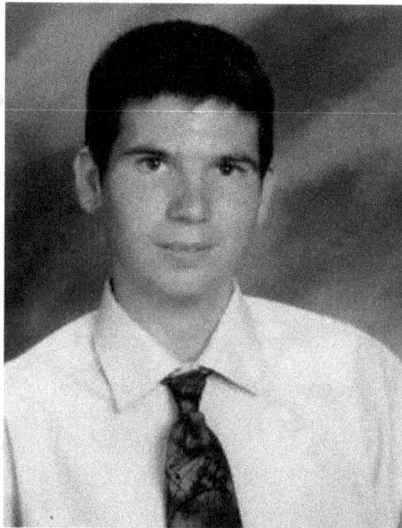

Figure 19. Jesse Gelsinger. Jesse's Intent

Most infants with OTC deficiency fall into a coma within 72 hours, suffering severe brain damage if they survive at all. Half do not live beyond their first month, and among those who do, half will not reach their fifth birthday.

Jesse's case was different. He had a partial form of OTC deficiency, a condition known as somatic mosaicism, which meant the mutation affected only some of his cells. This allowed him to manage the disorder through an arduous regimen of medication and a strictly controlled low-protein diet. But this management came at a cost: every meal was a calculated risk, every breath a delicate balance between survival and catastrophe. Ammonia levels in his bloodstream were a constant threat, ready to spike at the slightest misstep.

His cells, lacking the crucial enzyme needed to process ammonia, were constantly on the brink of being overwhelmed by this invisible poison. As a result, the Gelsinger household became a fortress of vigilance. Every gram of protein Jesse consumed was meticulously measured; every moment was shadowed by the specter of metabolic collapse.

His parents lived in perpetual readiness, always bracing for the possibility of an emergency. Paul Gelsinger, Jesse's father, bore the emotional scars of countless nights spent in hospital waiting rooms, his son's life hanging in the balance.

"Jesse battled for his whole life long," Paul said, his voice thick with emotion as he described their long journey. The strain of constant worry was etched into the lines of his face, a testament to the toll of loving a child with a life-threatening disorder.

Yet Jesse refused to let his condition define him. Despite the Herculean task of managing his health, taking nearly 54 pills daily, and adhering to an unforgiving diet, he lived with remarkable resilience. He pursued friendships, hobbies, and dreams for the future with a determination that belied the fragility of his health. For Jesse, these challenges were hurdles to overcome, not barriers to living.

But it wasn't always easy. Paul later recounted in *Jesse's Intent* how his son struggled at times to maintain the discipline required to manage his condition. He explains that " It took him nearly dying to wake him up."

On December 22, 1998, what began as an ordinary afternoon for Jesse Gelsinger and his family quickly spiraled into a medical emergency. When his father arrived home, he found Jesse curled up on the couch, pale and visibly shaken, with a close friend by his side. Jesse was vomiting uncontrollably, unable to keep down his medications; a critical situation for someone whose life depended on carefully managing his ammonia levels.

Alarmed, Paul Gelsinger immediately consulted with Jesse's pediatrician and specialist. It became clear that this was beyond anything they could handle at home. Jesse's ammonia levels had surged to six times the normal range, a life-threatening escalation that demanded immediate hospitalization.

Two days after Christmas, during a heartfelt conversation about Jesse's struggles, his father likened his situation to being stuck in a tree, unsure whether he would safely climb down or fall. That evening, Jesse called his father in distress, saying, *"Dad, I fell out of the tree."*

He was once again vomiting uncontrollably. Paul rushed back to the hospital, where the situation took a terrifying turn. As tremors overtook Jesse's body and he stopped responding altogether, panic gripped the room. Paul whispered urgently to his wife about their son's deteriorating condition just as medical personnel declared a code blue. They were swiftly removed from the room as doctors intubated Jesse and moved him into intensive care.

For two agonizing days, Jesse lingered in an induced coma while doctors fought to stabilize him. His weight had plummeted to 97 pounds, down from a healthy 120, and his previous medications were no longer sufficient to control his ammonia levels. Finally, on Thursday morning, the new medications arrived. Administered through gastrointestinal feeding, these treatments began to lower Jesse's ammonia levels within 24 hours.

As he regained consciousness, his first action was both mundane and profoundly reassuring: he gestured for someone to change the television channel, a small but unmistakable sign of his return to himself.

Later, in April of 1999, Jesse had recovered enough to learn about an experimental clinical trial at the University of Pennsylvania that aimed to treat ornithine transcarbamylase OTC deficiency using gene therapy. When he heard about it, something shifted in him — a spark of hope ignited in his eyes.

For Jesse, this wasn't just an opportunity for personal relief; it was a chance to contribute to something far greater than himself. The idea of helping others who shared his condition gave him a sense of purpose that transcended his own struggles. Paul, Jesse's father, recalled the moment with bittersweet clarity. He explains that it became a focal point. *The focal point* in Jesse's life, the hope in his son's voice, still echoes in his memory.

The science behind the trial was as bold as it was intricate. They planned to use an adenovirus, a common cold virus stripped of its harmful genes, as a delivery system for healthy genetic material. This was no ordinary virus.

It was a viral vector that had been re-engineered into a molecular courier capable of infiltrating liver cells and delivering a functional copy of the gene responsible for producing the enzyme Jesse's body lacked. This viral vector would carry a healthy copy of the gene. These viral vectors would infiltrate Jesse's cells, theoretically enabling them to produce the crucial enzyme he lacked.

At the helm of this ambitious trial was Dr. James Wilson, a pioneer in gene therapy research and the lead investigator at the University of Pennsylvania. The trial's dual purpose was clear: first, to treat the deficiency; second, to evaluate the safety of this cutting-edge therapy for future applications.

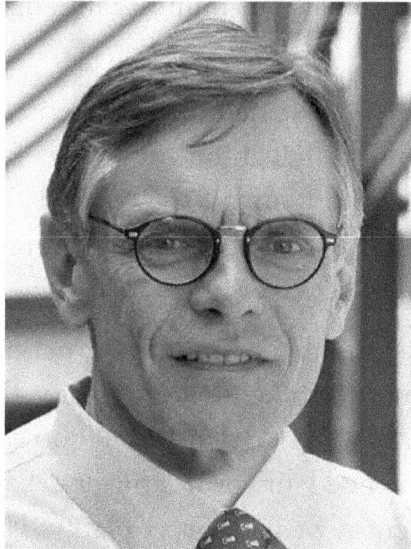

Figure 20. James Wilson. LouLou Foundation

Before committing to the trial, the Gelsinger family traveled from their home in Arizona to Philadelphia for an in-depth consultation

46

with Dr. Wilson and his team. The air buzzed with cautious optimism as medical jargon filled the room, words like *"vectors,"* *"enzymes,"* and *"clinical endpoints"* swirled around them. The doctors assured them that the risks involved were minimal. It was indicated that participants typically experienced only flu-like symptoms.

"The way they described it, this thing looked so safe," Paul recalled, his voice tinged with the bitter irony of hindsight. "Jesse was going to get the flu."

Bolstered by seventeen successful results from previous patients, the Gelsingers supported Jesse's decision to participate. Jesse underwent surgery to receive an infusion of a genetically engineered adenoviral vector carrying a corrected version of the gene. Initially, things seemed to be going as planned. The family felt a wave of relief, believing that Jesse had taken a step toward a better future.

Relief turned to alarm the next day when they received devastating news: Jesse's ammonia levels had doubled, and he was slipping into a coma. The situation escalated rapidly. Gelsinger vividly recalled the moment his world shattered with a single phone call.

When he finally reached Jesse's bedside, the sight that greeted him was beyond his worst nightmares. Jesse's body had betrayed him in the most harrowing way imaginable. His ears and eyes were grotesquely swollen shut, leaving him unresponsive—a stranger in his own skin.

"He had swollen so much, we couldn't recognize our own son," Paul whispered, the horror of that moment etched into his soul.

For four agonizing days, Jesse's family kept vigil at his bedside, clinging desperately to hope as doctors worked tirelessly to save him.

The relentless beep of monitors and hiss of ventilators formed a cruel symphony in the background, punctuated by hushed whispers from medical staff and muffled sobs from loved ones. But despite every effort, Jesse's condition continued to deteriorate.

When doctors finally confirmed there was no sign of brain activity, the Gelsingers faced an unthinkable decision: *they had to let their son go.*

On September 17, Jesse Gelsinger became the first person publicly identified as having died in a gene therapy clinical trial. His death sent shockwaves across the world, a stark reminder of the razor's edge between breakthrough and tragedy.

Dr. Mark Batshaw, one of the trial's investigators, later reflected on Jesse's death with profound regret: "Not a day goes by that I don't think of Jesse Gelsinger and his family," he confessed, his voice heavy with regret.

Dr. James Wilson, who led the trial, carried a similar burden. He was haunted by the choices that led to this tragedy. "With what I know now, I wouldn't have proceeded with the study," he admitted years later. The excitement surrounding gene therapy's potential had blinded them to its dangers. "We were drawn into the simplicity of the concept. You just put the gene in," he reflected on the naivety of those words, which is now a bitter reminder of the complexity and danger they had overlooked.

The aftermath of Gelsinger's death was seismic. Investigations were started in earnest. The findings were damning. Deeper looks into the tragedy revealed glaring lapses in protocol that cast a harsh light on the ethical and procedural flaws in gene therapy research. Jesse should never have been included in the trial, as his elevated ammonia levels disqualified him as a candidate. Moreover, prior adverse effects in other participants had not been promptly reported.

Despite the tragedy, initially, Paul Gelsinger and his family were outspoken supporters of those involved, believing they were acting in good faith. However, this trust was destroyed when they learned that the information provided to them was misleading. It was found that preclinical animal studies had revealed risks, including fatalities, that were not disclosed in the informed consent documents provided to Jesse and his family.

The investigators downplayed the dangers, suggesting that Jesse's liver would regenerate and omitting any mention of animal fatalities during the research. It's clear that the consent process had not been truly informed; the Gelsingers felt misled about the efficacy of the treatment and the associated risks.

This realization led to a full congressional investigation into the practices surrounding gene therapy trials. The investigation revealed significant lapses in oversight and ethical conduct. It resulted in fines for the institutions involved totaling over a million dollars. The fallout was swift and far-reaching.

Gene therapy protocols underwent immediate reevaluation, leading to stricter oversight, more rigorous safety measures, and a renewed focus on ethical considerations in clinical trials. Federal oversight tightened dramatically as all gene therapy trials across the United States were temporarily halted. Funding from both federal agencies and private industry dried up almost overnight, casting a shadow over what had once been one of medicine's most promising frontiers. The scientific community was forced to confront the uncomfortable reality of its ambitions.

~~~

In the wake of Gelsinger's death, the field entered what many would later call its *"silent era."* Once heralded as the vanguard of medical innovation, gene therapy became stigmatized. A "black label" in the eyes of both science and the public. The fear of repeating past mistakes loomed large, and funding dwindled as many hesitated to explore this once-celebrated frontier of medicine.

Jesse's death revealed a sobering truth: before we could attempt to rewrite the genetic code, we needed to fully understand it. This realization coincided with one of the most ambitious scientific efforts in history, the Human Genome Project. Launched in 1990, this monumental endeavor aimed to map and sequence all 20,500 human genes, collectively known as the genome. It was a scientific undertaking of unprecedented scale.

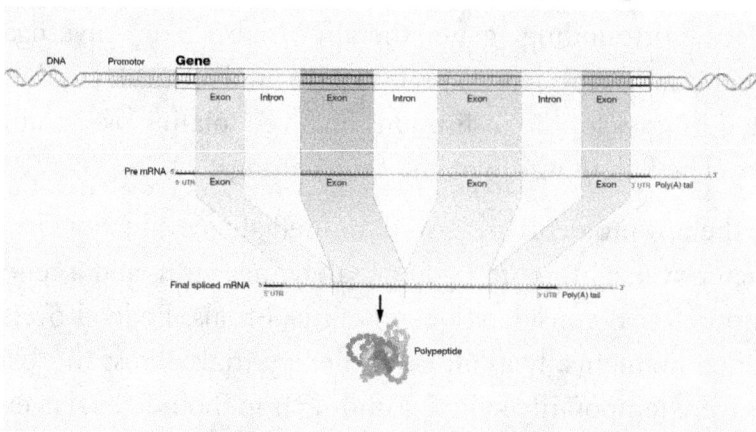

Figure 21. Gene. *National Human Genome Research Institute*

Behind the headlines of progress lay a more intricate and often messy reality. The project faced immense challenges: scientific, logistical, and ethical. From its earliest days, questions arose about how to ethically obtain DNA samples while ensuring donor anonymity. This was no ordinary research effort. The goal was not just to map genes but to create a reference genome that would serve as a foundation for understanding human biology and treating disease.

By 1996, clone libraries, collections of DNA fragments used for sequencing, were being distributed to laboratories worldwide. Yet, troubling revelations soon surfaced. Some of these libraries had been constructed without informed consent or oversight from institutional review boards, which are responsible for ensuring ethical compliance in research involving human subjects.

The situation grew even more complicated when rumors emerged that some DNA samples might have come from those directly involved in the project. This decision risked accusations of elitism and further blurred the lines of consent. Francis Collins, then director of the National Human Genome Research Institute, was deeply troubled. The fact that at least one donor's identity was known to the project team *and* that this donor was aware their DNA was being used violated the principle of anonymity that was supposed to underpin the project.

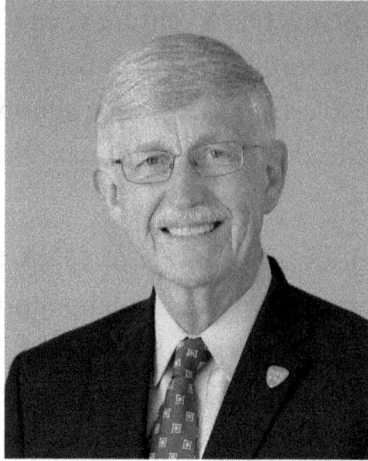

Figure 22. Francis Collins. National Institutes of Health, US DHHS

Determined to confront the ethical challenges head-on, Francis Collins and Aristides Patrinos, two key leaders of the Human Genome Project, took decisive action to rebuild trust and ensure the project adhered to the highest ethical standards. They devised a plan to create entirely new clone libraries under rigorous protocols. These libraries would employ a double-blind process: teams would not know the identities of donors, and donors would not know whether their DNA was ultimately used in sequencing efforts. This approach was designed to protect genetic privacy while preserving the integrity of the project.

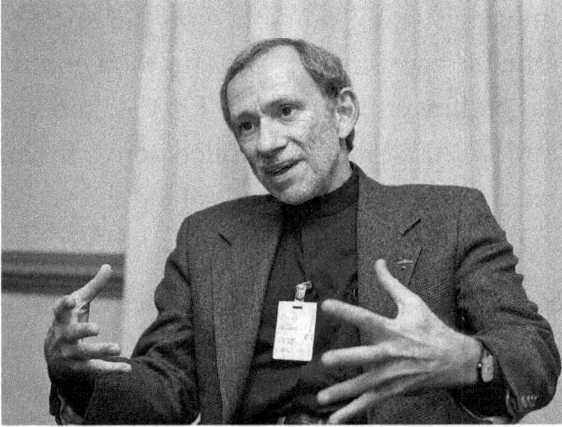

Figure 23. *Aristedes Patrinos. NASA*

To implement this plan, Pieter de Jong at Roswell Park Cancer Institute was tasked with constructing these new libraries. In March 1997, de Jong placed an advertisement in *The Buffalo News* seeking 20 volunteers willing to donate blood for research. Over the following weeks, volunteers met with genetic counselors, signed consent forms, and donated small blood samples. Each sample was anonymized. They were labeled only with a number, and two were randomly selected for use in creating clone libraries.

By August 1997, these new libraries were being distributed to labs worldwide, and Sanger's sequencing methods were put to the test. Among these libraries, one, *RP11*, emerged as particularly significant. It contained enough DNA fragments to span nearly the entire genome with minimal gaps and soon became central to the sequencing effort. In fact, RP11 ultimately contributed nearly 75% of the final genome sequence despite initial plans for a *"mosaic genome"* assembled from multiple donors

In laboratories scattered across the world, from the bustling halls of the National Institutes of Health in Bethesda to the serene research centers of Cambridge, teams embarked on the quest to map every nucleotide in the human genome. Eyes fixed on computer screens, they watched as endless streams of A's, T's, C's, and G's, those four letters that form DNA's alphabet, scrolled across their monitors in dizzying sequences. These cryptic codes held the secrets of human biology, waiting to be deciphered.

The air in these labs was thick with both excitement and exhaustion. Coffee cups littered desks like battle scars from countless late nights. Heated debates erupted over data interpretations, only to be punctuated by moments of triumph when another gene was successfully mapped. This was more than just science. It was a quest to understand the very essence of what makes us human.

Finally, in 2003, after more than a decade of relentless effort, a collective cheer echoed through research centers around the globe: the Human Genome Project was complete. The project successfully sequenced approximately 92% of the human genome. It focused primarily on the euchromatic regions, the gene-rich areas actively expressed in cells. These regions constituted about 90% of all gene-containing DNA. The remaining represented complex heterochromatic regions like centromeres and telomeres that resisted sequencing due to their intricate structures.

The sequencing of the human genome revealed that the approximately 3.1 billion nucleotides contained only about 20,000 to 25,000 protein-coding genes. To put this into perspective, imagine the genome as a vast library, its shelves stretching endlessly into the distance. Each book in this library contains 1,000 pages, with each page holding 3,100 letters, the average number of characters on a standard printed page. Representing the entire genome would require *one million such pages*. Stacked together, these books would form a tower taller than most skyscrapers.

Now, picture the part of this library that is dedicated solely to protein-coding genes, the parts of the genome that carry instructions for making proteins. It would be one small shelf with roughly 10,000 pages scattered across it. The rest of the library is non-coding DNA, often referred to as *"dark matter"*.

This dark matter is not "junk," as once thought; it plays critical roles in regulation and structure that we are only beginning to understand. These non-coding regions act as switches and scaffolds, influencing how and when genes are expressed, a complexity that helps explain how humans achieve such biological intricacy with relatively few coding genes.

If the sheer scale and visual of our genetic library feels overwhelming, that's because *it is*. In one striking example of visualization, an exhibit displaying just 1/1,000th of the human genome sequence—about three *million* letters— was displayed on a nearly 100-foot wall. Even at that reduced scale, the letters were so small they could barely be read without stepping in close to the wall.

The human genome is both vast and humbling. Its sheer size challenges our imagination while its sparse coding regions remind us how much we have yet to uncover about its mysteries. Completing the Human Genome Project marked a turning point in science and medicine. It provided an unparalleled roadmap for understanding human biology, a foundation upon which future discoveries could be built.

The lessons learned along this journey resonated deeply:

- *Progress must always be tempered by caution;*
- *Ambition must be balanced with ethical responsibility;*
- *and understanding must precede intervention.*

The completion of the Human Genome Project marked a turning point in our understanding of biology. For the first time, we had a comprehensive map of the human genome. But reading this map was only the beginning.

The real challenge lay ahead: translating this vast sea of data into meaningful insights about health and disease. It wasn't enough to know the sequence of our genes; we needed to understand how they worked, how they interacted, and how they could be used to improve lives. This shift, from reading the genome to applying its knowledge, sparked a new era in medicine.

CHAPTER 3

The Fundamentals of Genes and Gene Regulation

Suppose we unfurl the tightly wound DNA within just *one* of your cells. That slender thread would span nearly two meters if stretched to its entire length. Now, multiply that by the trillions of cells that compose your being. The combined DNA, pulled tautly, would become an astronomical cord, reaching from our blue planet to the incandescent surface of the sun and back again—not once, not twice, but a staggering 61 times.

This was once an untouchable world that was closed off from our understanding. But *now*, this vast library can be carefully read, copied, and changed using tools small enough to fit on a lab bench. As you read these words, researchers across the globe are unraveling the profound mysteries of DNA. They do this with the keen precision of master cryptographers, unlocking secrets that have long been hidden within the strands of our genetic heritage.

But the more we learn, the more we realize that DNA is not an isolated entity. Its story is interwoven with a complex web of interactions, a constant dance between genes and their environment. This understanding highlights the dynamic nature of DNA, which serves as more than just a static blueprint. It evolves in response to internal and external stimuli. And this, in essence, is the beautiful choreography at the heart of the Central Dogma.

The dogma is a carefully orchestrated flow of information from DNA to RNA to protein to phenotype, the very foundation upon which all life is built. Think of it this way: your DNA is like a master recipe book containing instructions for everything your body needs to function. *How, then, do these recipes translate into tangible proteins?*

~~❧~~

Imagine you are baking a cake using your master recipe book—a beautifully bound volume with detailed instructions for every single cake or protein your body requires to function. The cake we're baking is not just any cake; it influences everything about you, from the shape of your nose to how your heart beats. Let's say we need a specific cake, perhaps a fluffy, cloud-like angel food cake responsible for carrying oxygen in your blood or a sturdy, structural bundt cake that forms the scaffolding of your bones.

Your cell doesn't pull out the entire recipe book as it is stored safely in the nucleus of each cell. Instead, it identifies the correct recipe and makes a perfect photocopy on a separate card. This process is called transcription. Think of it as carefully rewriting the recipe from the master book onto a smaller, portable note.

This "recipe card" is made of messenger RNA or mRNA. Unlike the DNA recipe book, which is carefully guarded within the nucleus, the mRNA card is free to travel. It journeys out of the nucleus and heads towards the cell's bustling protein-making factories, the ribosomes.

Picture these ribosomes as vibrant kitchens filled with the gentle buzz of activity. Here, in the lively kitchen of the ribosome, a process called translation takes place. The mRNA strand is introduced to the ribosome, functioning like a recipe program. The ribosome reads the instructions and gathers specific ingredients called amino acids, which are the building blocks of proteins.

It assembles these amino acids individually, following the mRNA's coded instructions. This process is similar to a skilled baker adding flour, sugar, and eggs in the precise order and amounts needed. Once assembled, the newly formed protein, like a freshly baked cake, is ready to fulfill its specific function within the cell. But while the creation of the protein is a marvel of cellular engineering, it's just the prelude to a much richer story. What happens *next* is what truly defines its impact and role.

This is where phenotype becomes essential: it's all about how a protein interacts with its surroundings and shows up as a clear, observable trait. Think of the phenotype as the whole experience of enjoying a cake. It's not just about the ingredients that go into it. Instead, it's about how the world experiences that protein on a larger scale.

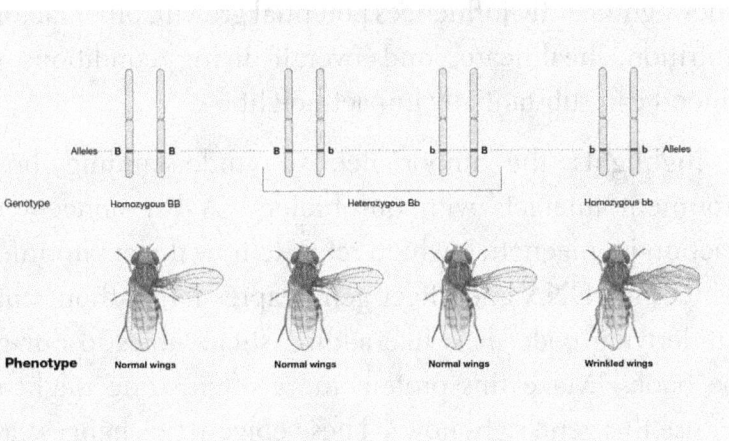

Figure 24. Phenotype. National Human Genome Research Institute

Take eye color as an example. The genes responsible for eye color act as the detailed cake recipe, guiding the creation of pigments such as the rich, warm honey of amber eyes, the piercing clarity of a cerulean blue, or the lush, deep greens of a forest canopy. These genes encode specific proteins. But the story doesn't end there; the interplay of multiple factors leads to our vast array of eye colors.

It's not merely the presence of these pigments but how they intertwine, like a symphony of colors. Just as a cake recipe combines various ingredients in precise proportions to create a delightful masterpiece, the quantity of each pigment produced can transform a subtle hazel into a radiant emerald. At the same time, the delicate structure of the iris itself, with its intricate patterns and textures, adds yet another layer of uniqueness.

Moreover, just as a single cake recipe can yield vastly different results depending on the baking conditions, such as altitude or humidity, our traits can also be expressed differently based on environmental influences. Take height as an example. Although genetics significantly influences potential growth, other factors such as nutrition, healthcare, and overall living conditions during childhood can substantially impact height.

This highlights the importance of understanding how our environment interacts with our biology. A key concept in this interaction is epigenetics, which refers to how the environment can influence our DNA and affect gene expression without changing the underlying code. It is like adding sticky notes to our genetic recipe book. "Make this protein more often," one might say, or "don't use this gene right now." These epigenetic changes can even be passed down to future generations.

Imagine if we could read these sticky notes, understanding the genetic code and how it's being interpreted in real time. *What secrets might we uncover about disease susceptibility, aging, or personality traits?*

This elegant system, from DNA to RNA to protein to phenotype, underlies every aspect of your biology. From the digestion of your food to the firing of neurons in your brain, every process depends on the precise and timely creation of these proteins. But as with many scientific "dogmas," the reality is far more nuanced and complex than initially thought.

The flow of information isn't always one-way. Certain viruses possess the remarkable ability to reverse the process, converting RNA back into DNA. This phenomenon, known as reverse transcription, challenges the traditional dogma of molecular biology, revealing a more fluid and adaptable system.

Discovered in the 1970s by David Baltimore and Howard Temin, reverse transcription converts RNA into complementary DNA, also called cDNA. Their work earned them the Nobel Prize in 1975 and improved our understanding of information flow. It also unlocked new possibilities in genetic engineering and therapeutic interventions.

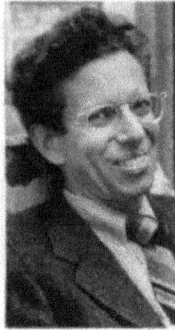

Howard Temin

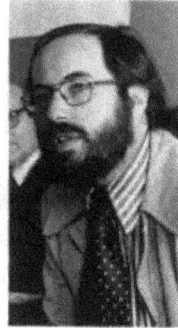

David Baltimore

***Figure 25**. Howard Temin and David Baltimore. Bioinfo & Unnati*

Retroviruses like HIV vividly demonstrate this process. These viral invaders carry their genetic information as RNA and deploy reverse transcriptase upon infecting a host cell. This enzyme acts as a molecular scribe, meticulously transcribing the RNA genome into DNA, which can then integrate into the host cell's genome, turning it into a viral replication factory.

The discovery of reverse transcription has profoundly impacted gene therapy and biotechnology. It enables the conversion of mRNA into DNA and the crafting of genes from RNA templates. This process can be likened to a molecular Xerox machine, creating DNA copies from RNA blueprints. It adds another layer to genetic storytelling, where the fleeting whispers of RNA are translated into the more enduring language of DNA, preserving and amplifying the message for generations of cells to come.

Picture a master scribe carefully translating the fleeting whispers of RNA into the more enduring language of DNA. This translation preserves the message and allows for its amplification and longevity. The scribe's quill moves with precision, each stroke ensuring that the therapeutic tale will be told for generations of cells to come.

Our understanding of genetics has evolved dramatically, revealing that our DNA is far more complex than once thought. Like an intricate tapestry, the genome weaves together protein-coding genes and vast stretches of DNA once dismissed as "junk." This non-coding DNA, we now know, produces RNA molecules that play critical roles in regulating gene expression.

Recall our genome library from before—a vast, ancient room walled with books, each book a gene. The protein-coding genes are like well-worn tomes, their stories frequently told. But interspersed among them are cryptic scrolls and hidden manuscripts, the non-coding regions, whose whispered secrets orchestrate the reading of the entire collection.

This library is not static but alive with activity. Transcription factors act as librarians, deciding which books to open and which to keep closed. They glide through the stacks, binding to specific DNA sequences like bookmarks, promoting or inhibiting the recruitment of RNA polymerase – the reader of our genetic texts. Like incantations in the margins, enhancers and silencers can influence gene expression from a distance, fine-tuning the cellular response to various stimuli.

At the heart of these intricate processes— DNA replication, RNA transcription, and translation into proteins—lie the true workhorses of the cellular world: enzymes. These protein structures act as biological catalysts, dramatically accelerating specific biochemical reactions essential for life. Suppose transcription factors are the librarians in our genetic library. In that case, enzymes are the skilled craftsmen who bring the library's contents to life.

~~

Enzymes, like master chefs in our cellular kitchens, expertly facilitate chemical reactions without being consumed themselves. They can speed up reactions by millions or even billions of times, enabling cells to carry out complex processes efficiently. Enzymes play a crucial role in many processes within our cells, from breaking down food to helping create DNA.

Just as a surgeon must understand both their tools and the patient's anatomy before a delicate operation, a deep comprehension of enzymes, DNA packaging, and cellular machinery is essential for grasping the power and potential of gene therapy. This foundational knowledge sets the stage for exploring the cutting-edge techniques and technologies that make genetic interventions possible.

First identified in the 1970s, restriction enzymes provide a striking example of nature's ingenuity. These proteins evolved in bacteria as a defense mechanism against invading viruses. They can identify and bind to specific DNA sequences. Once they locate their target, they act like highly specialized molecular scissors, cleaving both strands of the DNA double helix precisely at defined sites.

These molecular marvels, born from bacteria's ancient struggle against viral invaders, would soon become the scalpels of genetic engineering, allowing us to cut and paste DNA fragments with remarkable accuracy.

Picture a bustling bacterial cell, its DNA a tightly coiled blueprint of life. Suddenly, a virus injects its genetic material, threatening to hijack the cell's machinery and turn it into a factory for viral replication. But the bacterium isn't defenseless. It unleashes its secret weapon: restriction enzymes. These protein sentinels patrol the cellular landscape, their three-dimensional structure exquisitely tailored to recognize specific DNA sequences like a fingerprint.

When a restriction enzyme encounters its target, it's like a microscopic key sliding into an invisible lock. The enzyme's binding site embraces the DNA, its molecular fingers probing the grooves and ridges of the genetic code with the delicacy of a master safecracker. In a flash, the enzyme springs into action.

Its catalytic core cleaves through the DNA's sugar-phosphate backbone with the precision of a diamond cutter, leaving behind a clean, decisive incision. Some enzymes slice straight through both strands, leaving blunt ends as neat as a paper cut. Others create staggered incisions, producing sticky ends that dangle like frayed cosmic rope, their exposed bases yearning for complementary partners.

The applications of restriction enzymes are diverse. In agriculture, they help create crops with vibrant hues and enhanced flavors. They fortify plants against pests and harsh climates, turning fragile seedlings into resilient green warriors. In medicine, restriction enzymes illuminate the dark corners of our genetic makeup, allowing us to study disease-causing mutations. They pave the way for new gene therapies, offering hope to those burdened by inherited disorders.

But cutting is only half the story. What happens after we've precisely snipped a DNA strand?

That's where another class of molecules comes into play: DNA ligases. DNA strands stretch like delicate silk threads, carrying information. Suddenly, a strand snaps – a precise cut by the restriction enzymes. The DNA ligase is a molecular seamstress ready to mend the break with meticulous skill.

The ligase approaches the damaged site, its structure perfectly adapted to recognize the telltale signs of a DNA break. It settles into place, bridging the gap like a living suture. Then, in a flurry of atomic-level activity, it begins its work.

First, the ligase forms a bond with one end of the break. With one end secured, the ligase performs its signature move, its catalytic machinery whirring into action. It transfers the activated phosphate group to the other side of the break, forming a new bond and sealing the gap with molecular glue. In an instant, the DNA strand is whole again, its genetic message intact.

But what happens when it unravels?

This is where mutations come into play, those alterations in our DNA sequence that can ripple through an organism's entire being. Recall our ancient, sprawling genome library. Picture a clumsy librarian accidentally smudging a word here, tearing out a page there, or perhaps misplacing an entire volume. These genetic "typos" come in various forms, each with its own potential for chaos.

Point mutations are the subtlest of changes, like a single letter swap in a vast novel. A nucleotide might be replaced, inserted, or deleted, potentially altering the entire meaning of a genetic sentence. This can alter the codon—the three-nucleotide sequence that codes for an amino acid—potentially changing the protein's structure and function.

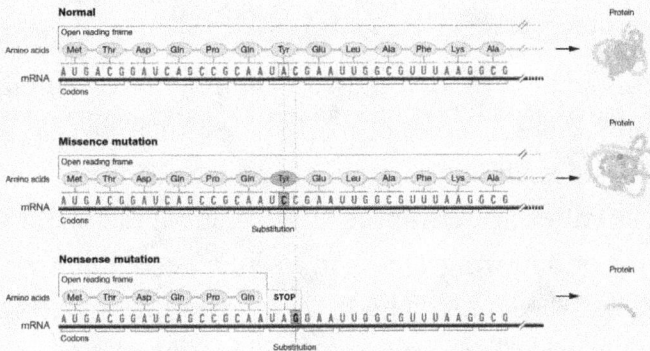

Figure 26. *Point Mutation. National Human Genome Research Institute*

Suppose we imagine DNA as a long string of colorful beads. A point mutation is like swapping one bead for another of a different color. Some of these changes are inconsequential, like swapping a red bead for another red bead- silent mutations that pass unnoticed through the cellular machinery. Other times, it can have dramatic effects, like in sickle cell, where a single bead swap turns normal, flexible red blood cells into rigid crescents that clog blood vessels like leaves in a gutter.

Missense mutations occur when a point mutation results in a codon that codes for a different amino acid. Scientifically, this can alter the protein's primary structure, potentially affecting its folding, stability, and function. Like a lock whose key has suddenly changed, the protein may no longer fit its intended purpose, leading to cascading effects throughout the cell.

On the other hand, nonsense mutations are abrupt full stops in the genetic narrative. They introduce a premature stop codon, scientifically known as a termination codon. This results in a truncated protein that is often non-functional. It's as if a book

67

suddenly ended mid-sentence, leaving the reader bewildered and the story incomplete.

Insertions and deletions, or indels, add another layer of complexity. Scientifically, if the number of nucleotides isn't divisible by three, it causes a frameshift, altering all subsequent codons. This means that these mutations can shift the entire reading frame of the DNA, like inserting or removing a letter in a sentence. Suddenly, "The cat sat on the mat" becomes "Theca tsa ton them at" - a nonsensical jumble that bears little resemblance to the original message.

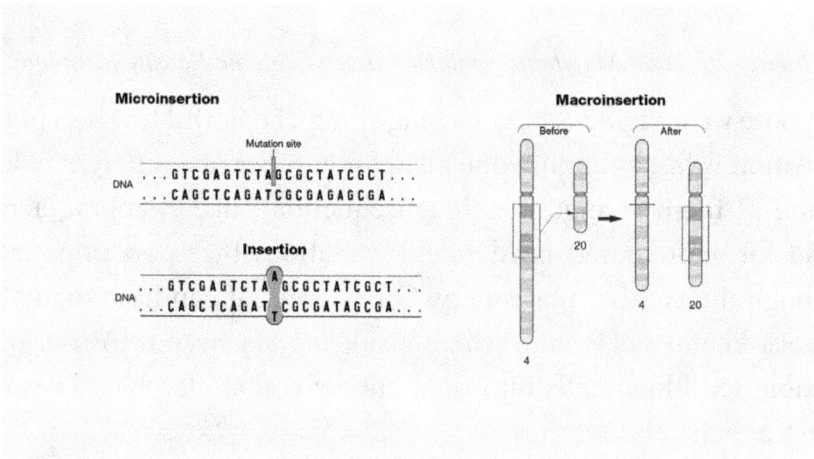

Figure 27. Insertion Mutation. National Human Genome Research Institute

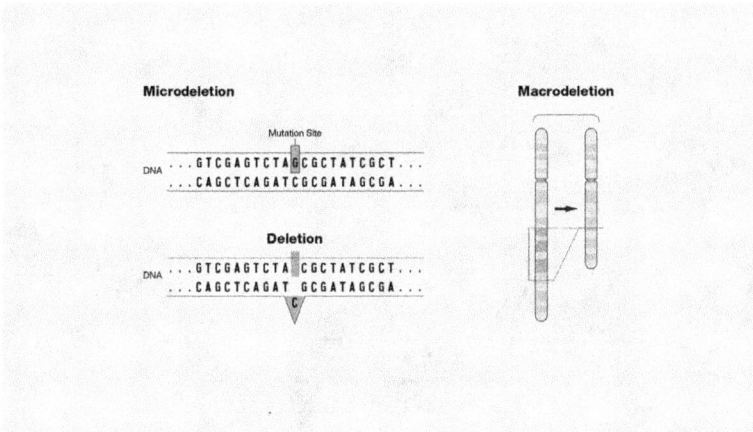

Figure 28. Deletion Mutation. National Human Genome Research Institute

Moving beyond single genes, we encounter more dramatic rewrites of our genetic story. Chromosomal mutations might flip and invert entire chapters, duplicate them, delete them entirely, or even paste them into a different book (translocation). The results can be devastating. It is as if someone is reorganizing entire chapters in a book - flipping them upside down, making multiple copies, removing them entirely, or moving them to a different book.

Copy number variations are like finding multiple copies of the same chapter in your favorite book. In the genome, extra copies of genes can lead to overproduction of specific proteins, potentially fueling the unchecked growth seen in some cancers. This can also lead to gene dosage effects, altering the amount of protein produced. Conversely, missing copies might leave the body without crucial cellular components.

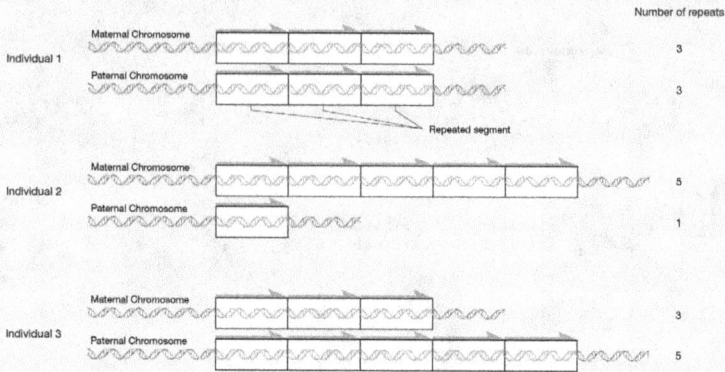

Figure 29. Copy Number Variation (CNV). National Human Genome Research Institute

Some mutations act like a genetic stutter, where a small DNA sequence is repeated repeatedly, expanding with each generation. A scratched record repeating the same phrase over and over. In biological terms, this "stutter" can grow worse over generations. This is seen in Huntington's disease, where an expanding CAG repeat in the huntingtin gene leads to toxic proteins that slowly poison nerve cells.

These mutations can arise from various sources, each contributing to the genetic diversity seen within populations. Our code is constantly under siege from a barrage of environmental influences, each leaving its mark on our molecular story.

For example, the sun's ultraviolet rays chisel away at our skin cells, shaping and reshaping the story written in our DNA. Radiation, both ionizing and non-ionizing, plays a role in this molecular makeover. X-rays and gamma rays are like scissors, potentially snipping our DNA strands. At the same time, UV light can cause letters to stick together and muddle the genetic message.

Alternatively, consider the chemical soup of modern life: pesticides, industrial emissions, and heavy metals, creating an environment where our DNA gets jostled and rearranged. These environmental mutagens are like clumsy editors, making unwanted changes to our genetic manuscript.

Specifically, pesticides might white out crucial letters, while heavy metals like lead, cadmium, and arsenic can crumple entire pages. Industrial pollutants act as overzealous highlighters, marking our DNA with potentially harmful additions. Even the air we breathe can harbor polycyclic aromatic hydrocarbons and volatile organic compounds, leaving smudges on our genetic blueprint.

Occasionally, these genetic missteps stumble upon a beneficial change. It's like accidentally discovering a shortcut while lost in a new city. A certain mutation, for instance, effectively locks the cellular door that HIV typically uses to gain entry. This anomaly offers a rare resistance to one of humanity's most persistent viral foes.

As a result, individuals with such beneficial mutations may gain an advantage in terms of survival and health within populations exposed to the virus. While mutations can be harmful or benign, they also play a critical role in adaptation in response to changing environments.

Understanding these changes is essential. By identifying the specific molecular errors that lead to diseases, we can develop targeted interventions—what some might call molecular Band-Aids to mend genetic issues or even comprehensive solutions to rewrite faulty genes. As we will explore in the upcoming chapters, gene therapy tools offer the possibility of correcting these errors at their source.

PART II
Rewriting Our Genetic Destiny

CHAPTER 4

The Tools That Are Rewriting Life

Victoria Gray, a 34-year-old mother of four from Forest, Mississippi, woke up each day not knowing if this would be the day her body betrayed her again. Sickle cell disease, a relentless genetic disorder, had transformed her blood into an adversary. Her red blood cells morphed into rigid crescents, resembling sickles. These distorted cells obstructed the flow of blood through her veins, creating painful blockages that starved her organs of the vital oxygen they desperately needed to function.

Each moment was a battle as her body endured the relentless toll of a condition that turned life-sustaining blood into a source of suffering. The pain was ruthless, a fiery torment that seared through her bones and joints, leaving her gasping and bedridden for days. Simple joys like attending her children's school events or even playing in the backyard were often beyond her reach. Victoria watched life pass her by, trapped in a cycle of hospital visits and opioid medications that barely kept the agony at bay.

While speaking at the Third International Summit on Human Genome Editing in London, Victoria said, "The pain I would feel in my body was like being struck by lightning and hit by a freight train all at once."

But in 2019, a glimmer of hope emerged. Victoria became one of the first patients to receive an experimental treatment using

CRISPR gene-editing technology. The procedure was grueling - her bone marrow cells were harvested, edited to produce healthy hemoglobin, and then reinfused into her body. For seven long months, Victoria endured the aftermath, her body slowly rebuilding itself from the inside out.

Then, one day, she felt a surge of energy she hadn't experienced in years. Tears of joy streamed down her face as she realized the "super cells," as she called them, were working their magic. The constant pain that had been her unwelcome companion for so long began to recede.

Today, Victoria stands tall, her eyes bright with newfound vitality. She holds down a full-time job, a feat that once seemed impossible. Weekends are filled with the sounds of cheering as she attends her children's football games and cheerleading events. Family outings, once a distant dream, are now a cherished reality.

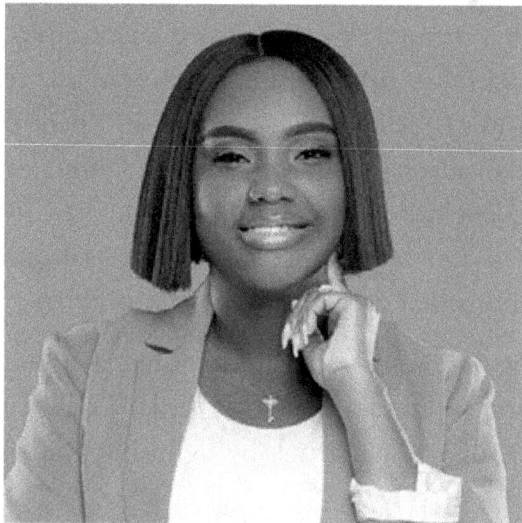

Figure 30. Victoria Gray. National Press Foundation

Victoria's transformation represents more than just a personal triumph; it is a testament to the relentless pursuit of healing. As we delve into the genetic tools used to change lives like Victoria's, we will see that they are transforming the practice of medicine and providing new hope to countless individuals and families impacted by disorders.

This hope is not unfounded. After decades of unraveling the mysteries of our DNA, we now stand at a pivotal moment in medicine. The journey that began with decoding the genetic blueprint has led us to an era where we can actively rewrite it.

The CRISPR-Cas9 system, which played a crucial role in Victoria's treatment, exemplifies this new frontier. It allows us to make precise changes to DNA within living organisms, enabling the correction of disease-causing mutations and even the insertion of missing genes. This technology has also shown promise in treating other conditions like hemophilia and certain cancers.

If earlier discoveries gave us the ability to read and understand the genetic code, CRISPR provides us with the power to edit it with unprecedented precision.

But what is CRISPR?

CRISPR, or Clustered Regularly Interspaced Short Palindromic Repeats, has ignited a firestorm in the scientific community. This novel gene-editing tool, originally a bacterial defense mechanism, has been ingeniously repurposed to modify DNA with unprecedented precision.

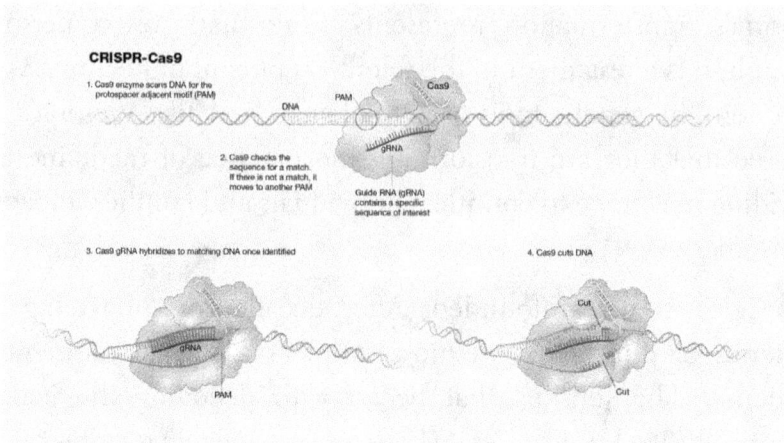

Figure 31. CRISPR. National Human Genome Research Institute

At its heart, CRISPR is nature's own genetic defense system, found in the microscopic world of bacteria and archaea. Picture these tiny organisms as fortresses, constantly under siege from viral invaders. When a bacterium survives a viral attack, it doesn't just celebrate its victory - it remembers.

It captures snippets of the virus's DNA, like taking snapshots of the enemy, and integrates them into its own genome within the CRISPR array. These captured sequences become a memory bank, allowing the bacterium to recognize and fend off future attacks from similar viruses quickly. But how does this bacterial defense system become a tool for genetic engineering?

The answer lies in two key components we have co-opted and refined in the CRISPR system. The first is guide RNA or gRNA, which acts like a GPS for genes. It is a short RNA sequence designed to match the target DNA within the genome. It functions like a molecular bloodhound that seeks out the specific DNA that requires editing.

The second component is the Cas9 enzyme, which serves as the system's workhorse. Think of it as a pair of incredibly precise molecular scissors. Once the gRNA has identified the target DNA, the Cas9 enzyme is guided to that location and makes a clean cut in the DNA strand, facilitating the editing process.

Introducing the CRISPR-Cas9 system into a cell is like sending in a highly trained special ops team. The gRNA locates and binds to its complementary DNA sequence in the genome - think of it as marking the target. Then, Cas9 follows the gRNA and cuts the DNA at the specified location, creating a precise double-stranded break.

But the story doesn't end there. Once the DNA is cut, the cell's natural repair mechanisms spring into action. It's like the body's construction crew rushing to fix a broken pipe. However, this repair process is often imperfect. It can introduce errors or, more importantly for us, allow the insertion of new DNA sequences. This is where the real power of CRISPR as a gene-editing tool comes into play.

What makes CRISPR so innovative is its precision and versatility. The gRNA can target virtually any DNA sequence, allowing for particular genetic modifications. It's like having a universal key that can unlock any door. Compared to earlier methods, CRISPR is a straightforward and cost-effective technique. It can be used in a wide range of organisms and cell types, including bacteria, plants, and human cells. This versatility makes CRISPR an invaluable tool for research and potential therapeutic applications.

The journey to CRISPR as a gene-editing tool spans several decades. It began in 1987 when CRISPR sequences were first observed in *E. coli*, though their function remained a mystery. In 2005, Francisco Mojica hypothesized that CRISPR is an adaptive immune system in bacteria. The real breakthrough came in 2012 when Jennifer Doudna, Emmanuelle Charpentier, and their teams demonstrated that CRISPR could be used for programmable gene editing.

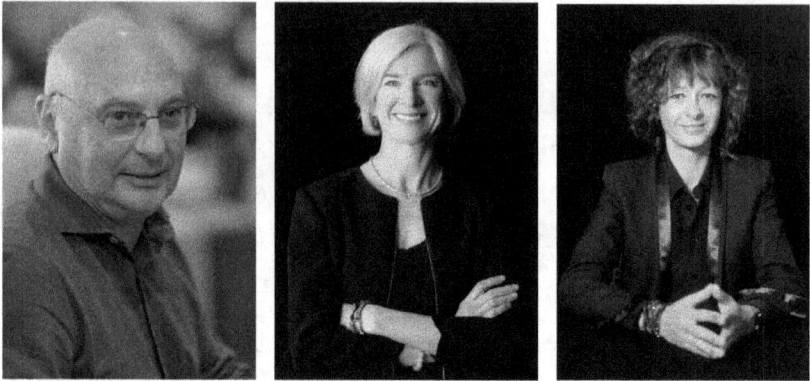

Figure 32. *Francisco Mojica, Jennifer Doudna, and Emmanuelle Charpentier. Manuel Castells from Flickr, Christopher Michel from Wikimedia Commons, Peter Bagde from the Kavli Prize*

This pivotal discovery accelerated research on human and nonhuman gene editing at lightning speed, paving the way for potential treatments for conditions like HIV, sickle-cell disease, and muscular dystrophy. It earned them the Nobel Prize in Chemistry in 2020.

Jennifer Doudna passionately promotes CRISPR's capabilities. She emphasizes its potential for healing and the ethical implications of such power. Doudna explains that gene editing allows for precise alterations to DNA within cells. She expresses her excitement about these advances: "It's been extraordinary to see how quickly CRISPR has taken off in labs around the world."

Within a few years, this once-futuristic technology has leaped from science fiction into practical application. CRISPR resonates through the scientific community, igniting a spark of inspiration in a new generation of researchers eager to push the boundaries of what is possible in genetic medicine. The once-insurmountable challenges posed by disorders are gradually being reframed as intricate puzzles waiting to be solved.

As with any powerful technology, CRISPR raises profound ethical questions that echo through the halls of science, igniting passionate debates. The ability to edit the human germline, making changes that could be passed down to future generations, has sparked intense discussions about safety, equity, and the very essence of what it means to be human.

~~♪

However, for all its promise, CRISPR faces a crucial challenge. A vehicle is needed to get inside the cells. So, the question is, how do we get the CRISPR-engineered gene where we need it?

The answer lies in an unexpected ally from nature's arsenal: biological vectors. These serve as "delivery trucks," carrying the therapeutic genes or gene-editing tools into the patient's cells. There are various types of vectors in the body, encompassing both viral and non-viral categories, each playing a crucial role in gene therapy and other medical applications.

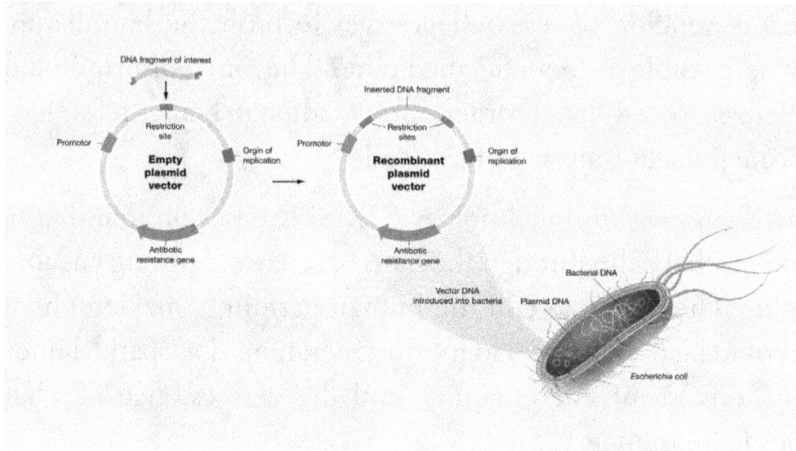

Figure 33. *Vectors. National Human Genome Research Institute*

The viral category of vectors has been engineered to safely transport genetic material without causing disease, opening up new possibilities for targeted therapy. By removing viruses' harmful properties, we have transformed them into Trojan horses capable of effectively delivering therapeutic genes into our cells.

The first vector we will discuss is adenoviruses. These have emerged as unlikely champions, transforming from common cold culprits into powerful allies in the battle against genetic disorders. We have repurposed these microscopic entities, once notorious for causing respiratory infections, into versatile tools.

Adenoviruses' appeal lies in their capacity to carry large genetic payloads, which distinguishes them among viral vectors. This expansive cargo hold allows us to package complex therapeutic genes, opening up possibilities for treating a wide array of previously deemed untreatable conditions. But it's not just their carrying capacity that makes adenoviruses so valuable; it's their ability to infect both dividing and non-dividing cells equally. This trait broadens their therapeutic potential to encompass a wide range of tissues and organs, making them ideal candidates for diverse medical applications.

The journey from pathogen to therapeutic agent begins with a process known as capsid engineering. This intricate procedure involves modifying the viral capsid proteins—the armor shielding the virus's material. We can fine-tune the virus's tissue tropism by altering these proteins and reprogramming its targeting system. This precision engineering allows the ability to direct the adenovirus to specific cell types with laser-like accuracy, ensuring the therapeutic genes reach their intended destinations while minimizing off-target effects.

Each modification to the viral capsid involves a calculated risk, venturing into uncharted territory where the distinction between healing and harm is often blurred. In this charged atmosphere of potential breakthroughs and daunting challenges, we turn our attention to another player in the viral vector arena—one that has been changing the field of gene therapy.

~●

The adeno-associated virus, or AAV, is a tiny marvel reshaping our approach to treating inherited conditions. Unlike its more notorious relatives, AAV operates with a subtlety that belies its enormous potential. These tiny viruses, measuring a mere 26 nanometers in diameter, about 3,000 times smaller than the width of a human hair, have become the heroes of gene therapy, offering hope through their minuscule payloads.

Initially discovered as contaminants in adenovirus preparations, AAVs were overlooked for years due to their seemingly harmless nature. However, as we peered deeper into their properties, we uncovered a treasure trove of characteristics that make them ideal candidates for gene therapy.

One of the most striking features is their ability to deliver genetic cargo with both precision and persistence. These viruses expertly navigate the body's cellular highways to drop off their therapeutic packages exactly where needed. Unlike viral vectors that trigger robust immune responses, AAVs slip past our body's defenses like silent messengers, delivering their therapeutic payload without such dramatic fanfare.

Though adverse reactions and immune responses are still very real possibilities due to these vectors, they are still more stealthy than others. This approach allows for long-term gene expression, a crucial factor in treating chronic genetic conditions. The potential of AAV-based therapies is vividly illustrated in the real-life story of Corey Haas.

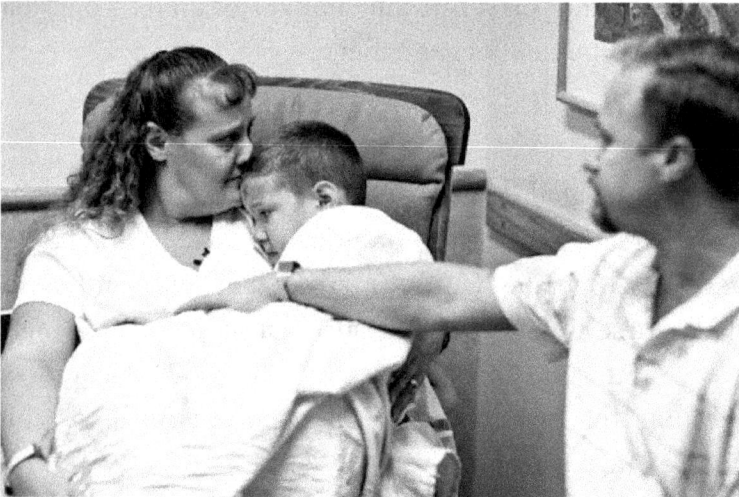

Figure 34. Corey Haas and Family. Stephen Voss

We meet 8-year-old Corey perched on the edge of an oversized chair in a dimly lit examination room at Children's Hospital of Philadelphia. His hands fidgeted with the hem of his shirt. Corey had never seen the world in full color. Born with Leber congenital amaurosis, a rare genetic disorder that causes blindness from birth or early childhood, his life had been a blur of shadows and muted tones. He navigated his world with the help of canes and assistance animals, his other senses heightened to compensate for what his eyes couldn't perceive.

But in 2008, Corey stood on the precipice of a treatment that promised to change everything. As the doctor explained the procedure, Nancy squeezed Ethan's hand, her knuckles white with tension. They had spent years searching for a solution, enduring countless doctors' appointments and experimental treatments. Each time, their hopes had been raised, only to be dashed again. But this time felt different.

Leber congenital amaurosis, caused by mutations in the RPE65 gene, prevents the retina from producing a crucial protein necessary for vision. The gene therapy proposed for Corey aimed to replace this defective gene, potentially restoring his sight.

The procedure itself was surprisingly quick. A tiny needle, loaded with millions of genetically modified viruses carrying healthy copies of the RPE65 gene, was carefully injected into Corey's right eye. As the needle withdrew, the room held its collective breath. Would this be the moment that changed everything, or just another disappointment in a long line of failed attempts?

The days that followed were a rollercoaster of emotions for the Haas family. Corey began to see colors he had never experienced before. Corey saw the world in vibrant color and sharp detail for the first time in his life. Shapes became focused, and the world around him burst into vivid life. He could navigate without assistance, play baseball, and engage in activities that were once beyond his reach. The AAV therapy hadn't just improved Corey's vision; it had opened up a new world for their son.

Corey's journey from darkness to light captured the world's attention, but it was not the first step in this field. It was the culmination of decades of research, trial, and error. The road to gene therapy's current achievements has been long and winding, marked by triumphs and setbacks.

In 2015, two pivotal studies published in *The New England Journal of Medicine* revealed both the promise and limitations of gene therapy for RPE65-associated LCA. While many patients experienced dramatic improvements in vision, the studies also documented ongoing degeneration of photoreceptor cells despite treatment, raising concerns about the long-term durability of the therapy.

Dr. Jean Bennett, who led Corey's trial, offered a nuanced perspective: "I could pick three patients in our trial and look at the data and say it doesn't work, and I can also pick another three and say it works fantastically."

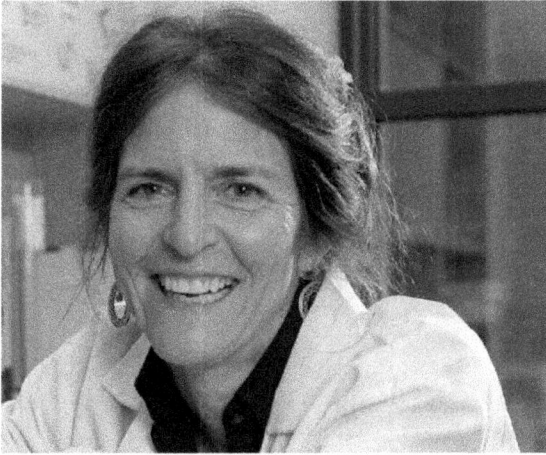

Figure 35. *Jean Bennett. United For Medical Research*

Dr. Eric Pierce, another pioneer in retinal gene therapy who worked with Dr. Bennett on the early clinical trial and is now at the Massachusetts Eye and Ear Infirmary, compared the trajectory of this field to that of penicillin.

"When it was introduced in the 1940s, not everybody responded, and we learned over time that we use different doses and routes of administration to treat different diseases. Should we have given up on penicillin? Call it bad because it didn't work on everyone the first time we tried it. We needed to learn to use it effectively and develop additional antibiotics to treat what penicillin doesn't. It will be the same story for gene therapy."

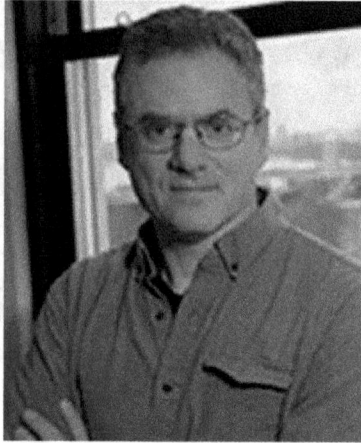

Figure 36. Eric Pierce. Harvard Ophthalmology Communications Office

Indeed, setbacks are part of progress. The studies highlighted that vector design and surgical techniques significantly influence outcomes. These challenges have spurred us to refine approaches rather than abandon them.

As Dr. Bennett aptly put it: "It would be naive to think that any drug is going to work perfectly all of the time. And it is also naive to think that we can immediately turn someone who is severely visually impaired into someone with 20/20 vision. We are still learning about the variables that determine success."

In 2017, Corey's treatment, now known as Luxturna, received FDA approval, marking it the first gene therapy approved in the U.S. for an inherited disorder. Corey's journey from darkness to light stands as a testament to the power of gene therapy and the relentless pursuit of scientific breakthroughs. It underscores the potential of these tiny viral vectors to bring about profound changes in patients' lives, transforming what was once a bleak prognosis into a future filled with possibilities.

This therapy may not yet offer a permanent cure for blindness, but its impact cannot be overstated. For example, Dr. Pierce feels these results are incredibly significant. He says, "People have been trying to develop treatments for LCA and related inherited blindness for 100 years. Nothing has ever worked before, and here are the first therapies that work. It's still a huge advance, but we must perfect it."

The journey continues as we explore new frontiers in treating blindness. Each step forward builds on decades of perseverance and innovation, bringing us closer to a future where inherited blindness may no longer define anyone's life story.

~

The versatility of AAVs extends far beyond ocular diseases, reaching into the complex realm of blood disorders. For individuals with hemophilia, life has long been a precarious balancing act, with the specter of uncontrolled bleeding casting a shadow over even the most mundane activities. But AAV-mediated gene therapy is rewriting this narrative, offering a glimpse of a future where hemophilia is not a life sentence but a manageable condition.

Imagine standing at the edge of a vast, intricate clockwork mechanism, its gears and levers stretching as far as the eye can see. This is the human body's clotting system, a marvel of biological engineering that springs into action at the first sign of injury. In a healthy individual, this mechanism whirs to life with breathtaking precision, each component playing its part in a life-saving symphony. But this finely tuned machine harbors a fatal flaw for those with hemophilia.

Picture a young boy, let's call him Alex, playing in the park. He trips and scrapes his knee - a minor incident for most children. Still, for

Alex, it's the beginning of a potentially life-threatening ordeal. As the first drops of blood appear, Alex's body desperately tries to activate its clotting cascade. But it's like an orchestra missing its conductor; the musicians are present, but without direction, they can't produce the harmony needed to stem the flow.

In Alex's case, it's Factor VIII that's absent, the hallmark of Hemophilia A. For others, like Jen, a teenager with Hemophilia B, it's Factor IX that's missing. These crucial proteins are the maestros of the clotting symphony, coordinating the complex dance of platelets and fibrin that form a stable clot.

Without them, Alex and Jen face a constant, invisible threat. Every bump, every fall, every seemingly innocuous injury carries the risk of uncontrolled bleeding. Worse still is the specter of internal bleeding: silent, insidious, and potentially crippling. Imagine the constant anxiety, the hyper-vigilance required to navigate a world where your own body can't be trusted to perform one of its most basic functions.

But now, picture a laboratory humming with activity. The process begins here, where we engineer AAVs to carry the genetic instructions for producing Factor VIII or IX. These viral vectors are then injected into the bloodstream, where they home in on liver cells with precision.

Inside the liver cells, this new code springs to life. Molecular machinery whirs into action, following the blueprint to produce the once-missing Factor VIII. It's as if a long-dormant assembly line has suddenly roared to life, churning out the very protein that Alex's body has craved since birth.

What makes this moment truly breathtaking is its potential for lasting change. Unlike the regular infusions that have punctuated

Alex's life, this single treatment could provide years, even decades, of protection. It's not just a temporary fix; it's a fundamental rewriting of Alex's biological script.

One particularly fascinating aspect of this research is the development of "codon-optimized" transgenes. These squeeze every drop of therapeutic potential from each successfully treated cell, maximizing the impact of the therapy. By tweaking the genetic code of the clotting factor genes, we can enhance their expression in liver cells..

The results of clinical trials have been published in *the New England Journal of Medicine.* Patients with severe Hemophilia B who received AAV gene therapy showed sustained production of Factor IX at levels that dramatically reduced or eliminated the need for regular factor infusions.

Patients who once lived in fear of every bruise now lead lives unburdened by the constant threat of bleeding. The need for regular infusions, a time-consuming and often painful reminder of their condition, fades away. It's as if a heavy chain has been lifted, allowing these individuals to step into a world of newfound freedom and possibility.

Activities that were once fraught with danger – playing sports, traveling, or even something as simple as shaving – suddenly become possible without the constant fear of a bleeding crisis. The psychological burden of living with a chronic, potentially life-threatening condition begins to lift, replaced by a newfound sense of freedom and normalcy.

But the story doesn't end with hemophilia. The success of AAV gene therapy in hemophilia has flung open doors that were once thought impenetrable, revealing vistas of hope for a myriad of other blood conditions. We are now exploring similar approaches for conditions like sickle cell disease, beta-thalassemia, and even certain types of anemia.

Yet, as with any journey into uncharted territory, the path ahead is fraught with challenges that loom like storm clouds on the horizon. In quiet hospital rooms and bustling research centers, long-term safety studies are underway. Patients who received these therapies years ago are closely monitored, their every blood test scrutinized for signs of unexpected complications. The question that hangs heavy in the air, unspoken but ever-present: *Will the benefits of these treatments stand the test of time?*

~

Another development is helper-dependent adenoviral vectors, often called "gutless" vectors. By stripping away all viral genes except those essential for packaging, these vectors can carry larger genetic payloads with significantly reduced immunogenicity. These gutless vectors aren't just delivery vehicles; they're precision-guided missiles in the war against diseases.

With their significantly reduced immunogenicity, they offer the tantalizing prospect of repeated treatments without triggering a devastating immune response. It's as if they've found a way to slip past the body's defenses undetected. This opens new avenues for delivering complex therapies requiring more extensive genetic information.

There are many other potential vectors that are not related to adenoviruses that are also being studied and used. Imagine a viral vector with the ability to carry an extensive payload of therapeutic genes, navigating the intricate pathways of the nervous system with an innate precision honed by millions of years of evolution. This is the herpes simplex virus or HSV, a viral vector with an appetite for genetic cargo that dwarfs its competitors.

Picture standing before a vast library of information. Most viral vectors can carry only a few slim volumes, but HSV strides in like a giant, capable of hoisting entire shelves of books, with a genome capacity of up to 150 kilobases. Complex genetic constructs and multiple therapeutic genes can all be packaged within its expansive confines.

Its natural neurotropism – the ability to preferentially infect neural tissue – means that HSV can deliver its cargo directly to the cells that need it most, minimizing off-target effects and maximizing therapeutic potential. It is like a built-in GPS, allowing it to navigate the intricate pathways of the nervous system with a precision that seems almost magical.

～

As we move beyond the realm of HSV, we encounter the intriguing world of retroviruses and lentiviruses. These can weave their genetic material directly into the fabric of the host cell's genome. The potential of this is staggering, but so are the risks. This power to alter the genome permanently is a double-edged sword, offering the promise of long-lasting therapeutic effects but also carrying the risk of unintended consequences.

At the Children's Hospital of Philadelphia, a young Emily Whitehead sat on her bed, her small legs dangling over the side. Her parents, Tom and Kari, gently stroked their daughter's hair, trying to mask their worry. Emily's once vibrant blue eyes now seemed dull, her movements slow and unsteady; telltale signs of the acute lymphoblastic leukemia that had been slowly robbing her of her childhood.

The doctor entered the room, his presence filling the space with a mixture of hope and apprehension. In his hands, he held a small vial containing what looked like clear liquid, but within this unassuming fluid lay Emily's chance at a new life.

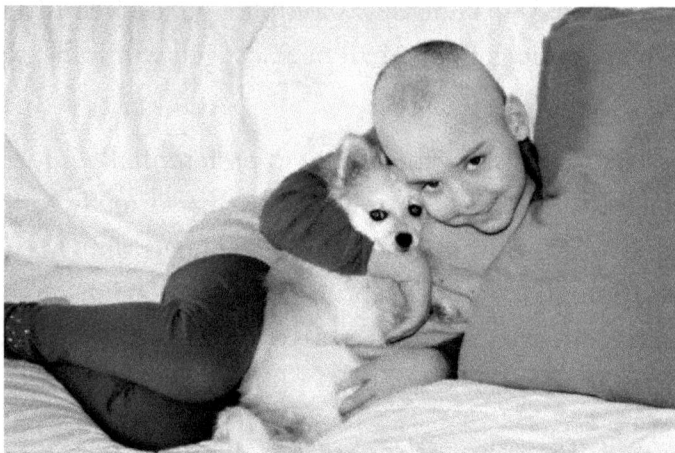

Figure 37. Emily Whitehead. Emily Whitehead Foundation- Activate the Cure® for Childhood Cancer

At just 6 years old, Emily became the first pediatric patient to receive CAR T-cell therapy for acute lymphoblastic leukemia. This treatment used a lentiviral vector, a type of retroviral vector derived from HIV-1. These vectors have a unique ability to infect non-dividing cells, making them particularly useful for targeting a wide range of cell types. In Emily's case, the lentiviral vector was used to deliver genetic instructions to her T-cells, reprogramming them to recognize and attack cancer cells.

The use of lentiviral vectors in Emily's treatment showcased their potential for stable gene transfer. Unlike some other gene delivery methods, lentiviral vectors can integrate their genetic payload into the host cell's genome, potentially providing long-term therapeutic effects.

Yet, this same power that offers such hope also casts a shadow of concern. The integration of viral DNA into the host genome is a double-edged sword, a high-stakes gamble where the potential rewards are matched by equally significant risks. One of the primary concerns has been the risk of insertional mutagenesis, where the integration of the vector into the host genome could potentially disrupt normal gene function or activate oncogenes.

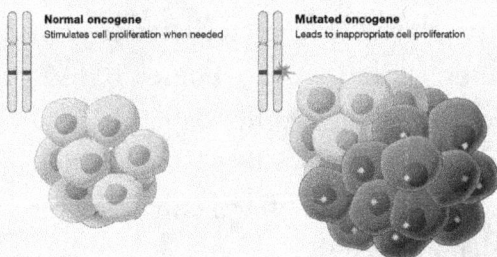

Figure 38. Oncogenes. National Human Genome Research Institute

Oncogenes are like light switches in your cells that control growth and division. Normally, these switches are turned off or only activated when needed. However, sometimes these switches can get stuck in the "on" position due to gene mutations. When oncogenes are activated, it's as if someone flipped the light switch and left it on permanently. This causes cells to grow and divide uncontrollably, which can lead to cancer.

This risk looms large, a reminder that in tampering with the genome, we may disrupt the delicate balance of gene expression. It's a tightrope walk between cure and complication, where a misstep could lead to the activation of oncogenes, potentially trading one disease for another.

To mitigate these risks, self-inactivating vectors were developed. These modified vectors have deletions in the viral promoter and enhancer elements, reducing the likelihood of unintended gene activation. More work remains to be done in solidifying the safety of these treatments.

~~♪

Our journey through the viral vector landscape takes another turn as we encounter alphaviruses. These RNA viruses are the overachievers of the viral world, capable of inducing protein expression at levels that boggle the mind. In the realm of cancer immunotherapy, alphaviruses offer a tantalizing possibility: turning cancer cells into their own worst enemies.

In 2017, within the sterile yet charged atmosphere of Duke University, a phase I clinical trial was underway. We were harnessing the power of an attenuated poliovirus to confront one of the most formidable foes in medicine: recurrent glioblastoma, an aggressive and often fatal form of brain cancer. The air was thick with anticipation as they tested this novel approach, which aimed to infect tumor cells and trigger a robust immune response against the relentless cancer.

Among the patients enrolled in this pioneering trial was Stephanie (Lipscomb) Hopper, a brave 20-year-old who had been battling glioblastoma since her diagnosis in 2011. As she sat in her hospital room, the weight of her journey hung heavily in the air. After enduring conventional treatments that had ultimately failed her, Stephanie found herself at a crossroads, ready to embrace an experimental therapy that offered a glimmer of hope.

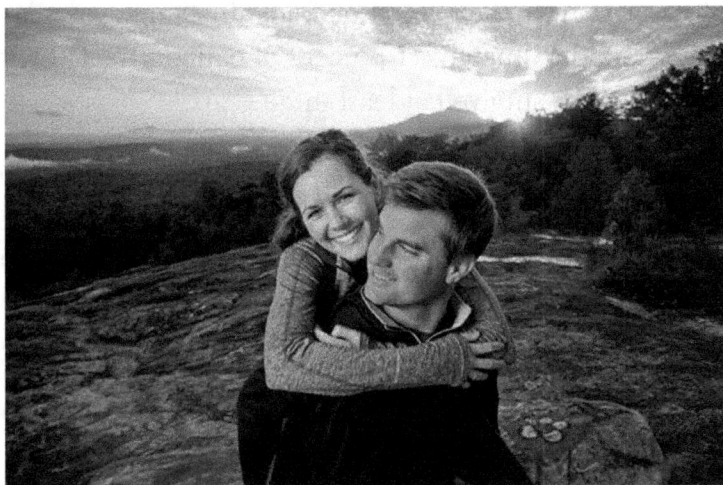

Figure 39. Stephanie (Lipscomb) Hopper. Jared Lazarus and Duke Neurosurgery

As the infusion began, there was a cool sensation coursing through her veins. The clear liquid flowed steadily into her body, carrying with it not just the engineered virus but also the hopes of countless researchers and families who believed in this approach. It was as if she were being infused with possibility itself.

Days turned into weeks after the treatment. The tumor began to shrink—slowly at first, then more rapidly—as if it were retreating from an unseen army unleashed within her body. The modified poliovirus was doing its job; it was attacking the cancer cells while simultaneously rallying Stephanie's immune system to join the fight.

The Duke University team compared their 61 volunteers who received this therapy to similar past patients who did not receive the treatment. Among those historical controls, all but one patient died after an average of 11 months, with only 14 percent surviving two years after diagnosis and a mere 4 percent alive three years later. In stark contrast, approximately 21 percent of patients treated with the modified poliovirus survived at least three years.

With each follow-up appointment, she could feel the weight of despair lifting as she learned about her progress. The dual action of directly assaulting cancer cells and stimulating the immune system mirrored what we hoped to achieve with alphavirus-based treatments. This is a tantalizing glimpse into a future where viruses could be allies in the battle against cancer.

Years later, Stephanie remained cancer-free, defying all odds and proving wrong those who believed recurrent glioblastoma was an unwinnable battle. Her case became a beacon of hope for others facing similar diagnoses, demonstrating that innovative viral therapies could transform tumors into targets for the immune system.

However, this inspiring journey took a poignant turn. On March 26, 2020, Stephanie Hopper passed away at the age of 28, eight years after undergoing the poliovirus treatment. The therapy granted her eight additional years of life, which she embraced fully. During this time, she married her longtime soulmate, Matthew Hopper, in 2018 and completed nursing school, dedicating herself to helping others as a nurse at Prisma Health Greenville Memorial Hospital.

Duke's Dr. Annick Desjardins, who was Stephanie's neuro-oncologist, remarked on Stephanie's profound impact in an article by Duke: "From the first day Stephanie and I discussed the genetically modified poliovirus, and the fact that she would be the first human treated with it, she understood what it meant to science and glioblastoma patients. Stephanie took her role very seriously. She dedicated herself to helping others, not just glioblastoma patients like her, but every patient who had the chance to have her as a nurse, sometimes to the detriment of her own health. It was a privilege to know her. Stephanie's energy and grace will continue to push me in our quest to conquer this tumor." Her legacy continues to inspire both patients and medical professionals alike.

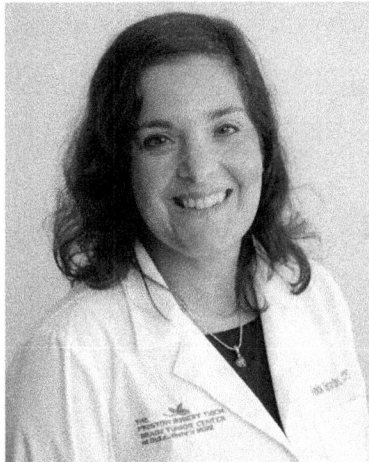

Figure 40. Annick Desjardins. Duke Neurosurgery

Tom O'Donnell, another brain cancer patient at Duke, expressed gratitude for having met Stephanie through their shared struggle: "It was my brain tumor that allowed me to meet Stephanie, and for this I am grateful. She showed us what brave looks like. She blazed the path for the rest of us to follow. We will continue to fight the good fight and push relentlessly forward toward the cure."

Stephanie's journey exemplifies resilience and hope in the face of adversity, reminding us all of the potential that innovative treatments hold in transforming lives and advancing cancer research. Each viral agent represents a vessel, ready to carry us into new territories of treatment and cure.

In this microscopic arena, we are not mere observers, but active participants in the ongoing evolution of life. We wield tools that nature has perfected over billions of years, repurposing them to heal, to cure, and to redefine the limits of medical science. It's a dance of molecular precision, where the line between friend and foe blurs as we harness the very mechanisms that viruses use to cause disease and turn them into powerful allies in our quest for health.

Yet, as we venture into this brave new world, we must navigate treacherous waters. The challenges are as numerous as they are daunting.

How do we ensure the safety of these viral vectors? How do we target them precisely to affected cells without causing collateral damage? How do we overcome the immune responses that our bodies naturally mount against these viral invaders?

~♪

Viral vectors have long been the virtuosos of gene delivery. But alongside these viral virtuosos, a new movement is emerging. Non-viral methods are appearing with reduced immunogenicity and streamlined production processes. At the forefront of this non-viral orchestra are lipid nanoparticles.

Imagine these as tiny bubbles, no larger than a thousandth of a human hair's width, yet carrying within them the power to rewrite our code of life. Their outer shell, a carefully orchestrated arrangement of lipids, forms a protective cocoon around the delicate genetic cargo within. This lipid bilayer is not just a simple barrier; it's a dynamic, responsive entity, adapting to its environment like a chameleon changes colors.

The lipid nanoparticles glide through this hostile environment with remarkable stealth. Their surface, adorned with polyethylene glycol or PEG molecules, creates an invisibility cloak, allowing them to evade detection by the immune system. They navigate the treacherous waters of the bloodstream and shield their precious payload from degradation.

Upon reaching their cellular destination, the lipid bilayer senses the change in its surroundings and begins to fuse with the cell membrane. As the fusion completes, the LNPs release their precious cargo into the cellular cytoplasm with the finesse of a magician revealing their grand illusion.

Once inside, the delivered nucleic acids—be they mRNA, siRNA, or plasmid DNA—begin their own function. mRNA molecules race to the ribosomes, conducting the synthesis of therapeutic proteins. siRNAs seek out and silence harmful genes with surgical precision. Plasmid DNA, the most ambitious of performers, makes its way to the nucleus, where it can integrate into the cell's genome, potentially offering long-term therapeutic effects.

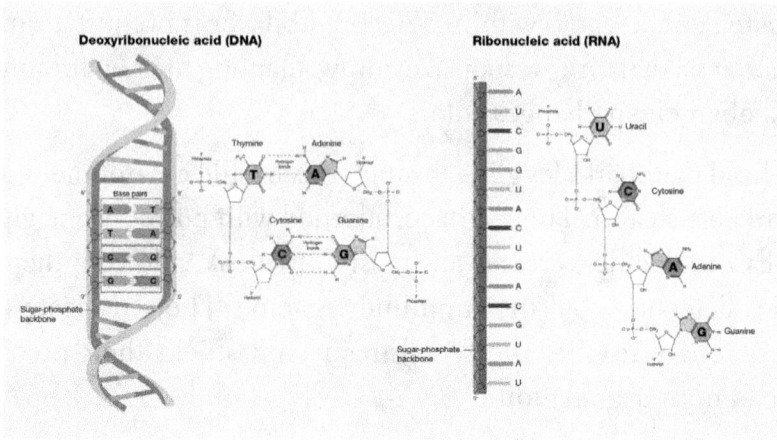

Figure 41. Nucleic Acids. National Human Genome Research Institute

This efficient delivery system has opened up new possibilities for gene therapy, allowing for the introduction of large and complex genetic instructions that were once thought impossible to deliver without the help of viruses.

~~

The success of mRNA vaccines against COVID-19, delivered via lipid nanoparticles, has catapulted this technology into the spotlight. Now, we are exploring these for treating genetic disorders, cancer, and even as tools for precise genome editing. Another new player has emerged, adding intricate melodies to our growing symphony of therapeutic possibilities.

The discovery of RNA interference, RNAi, in 1998 by Andrew Fire and Craig Mello was like uncovering a hidden symphony within our cells, a revelation that would forever change the landscape of molecular biology. Their work, which earned them the Nobel Prize in 2006, unveiled a natural cellular process that could silence specific genes. This offers promising strategies for treating various conditions, from genetic diseases to cancer. The discovery opened a new chapter in molecular biology and laid the foundation for a new class of therapeutics.

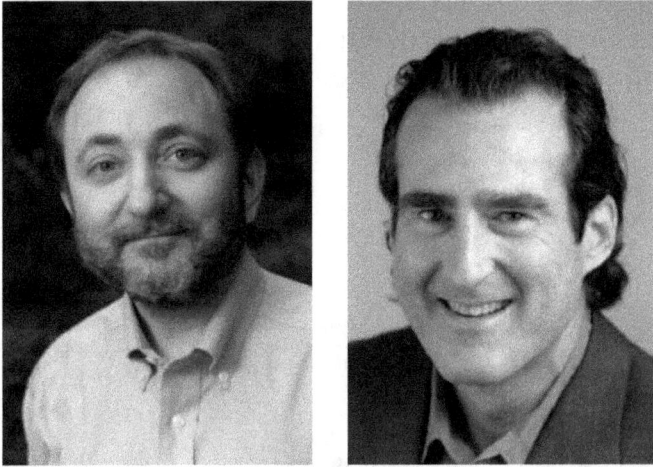

Figure 42. Andrew Fire and Craig Mello. Nobel Prize Outreach

Picture a world where we could fine-tune the human genome like a master violinist adjusts their strings. This is the promise of RNA therapeutics. Unlike the permanent alterations of DNA-based therapies, RNA approaches offer a more nuanced and potentially safer alternative. It's as if we've discovered a genetic dimmer switch, allowing us to modulate gene expression without the risks associated with permanently rewriting our code.

Today, we understand RNA's versatility as a tool for modulating expression without the inherent risks associated with permanent genetic changes. This realization sparked a paradigm shift in the approach to therapies. While DNA-based gene therapies aimed to correct faulty genes by altering the DNA sequence, RNA-based approaches offered a more nuanced and potentially safer alternative.

The science behind RNA therapies is both intricate and compelling. RNA is the essential messenger that transmits genetic instructions from DNA to the cellular machinery responsible for protein synthesis. Small interfering RNAs act like molecular scissors, precisely snipping away at malfunctioning messenger RNA, which contributes to disease.

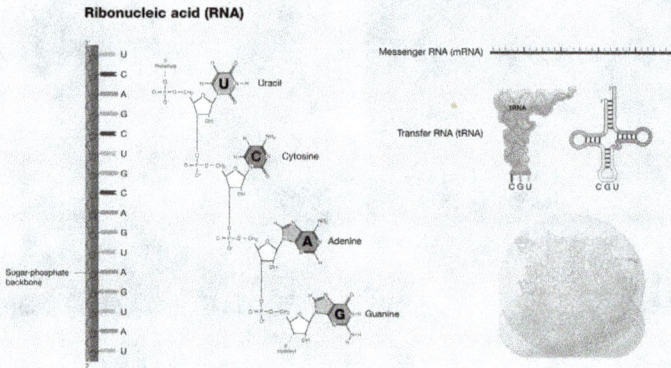

Figure 43. RNA. National Human Genome Research Institute

These siRNAs are skilled editors, meticulously excising unwanted passages from the genetic score of life. Their exquisite specificity allows them to target and degrade only the mRNA sequences that match their own, triggering a cascade that silences the problematic gene.

Antisense oligonucleotides play a different tune in this RNA ensemble. These short, synthetic nucleic acid sequences are the conductors of our cellular symphony, modulating gene expression by binding to complementary RNA sequences. With the wave of their molecular baton, they can influence splicing patterns, block protein translation, or induce the degradation of target RNAs. It's a versatile toolkit that allows us to fine-tune genetic expression with unprecedented precision.

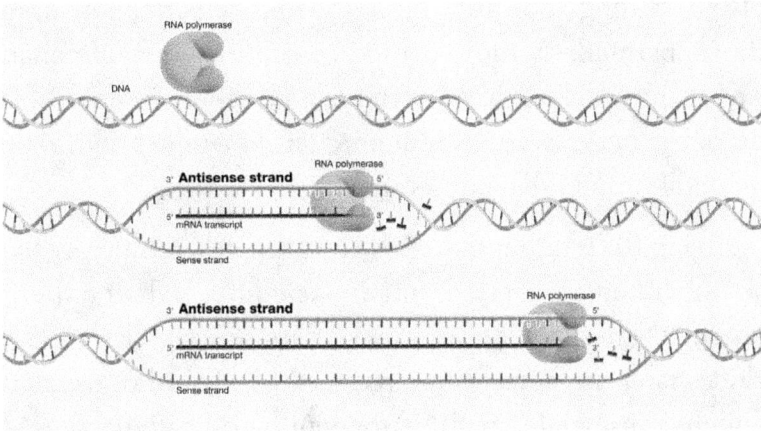

Figure 44. Antisense. *National Human Genome Research Institute*

Perhaps the most innovative movement in this non-viral composition is messenger RNA or mRNA, therapeutics. By delivering mRNA that encodes therapeutic proteins, we can induce a temporary but powerful production of beneficial proteins without altering the underlying genomic code. It's as if we're handing our cells a new sheet of music, allowing them to become transient protein factories that follow our carefully crafted melody without altering their repertoire permanently.

As our understanding deepens, we're discovering new instruments in the form of long non-coding RNAs, lncRNAs. Once dismissed as "junk RNA," these molecules are now recognized as important regulators of gene expression, particularly in cancer. They're like the hidden counterpoint in a complex fugue, subtly influencing the overall composition of cellular function.

As we reach the crescendo of our RNA exploration, a new frontier emerges: ADAR, or adenosine deaminase acting on RNA editing. This RNA editing tool allows for the direct correction of RNA mutations, particularly those caused by single-nucleotide changes. It's like having a master copyist who can correct a single misplaced note in our genetic score, introducing safer therapies with reduced likelihood of unintended consequences.

By modifying RNA rather than DNA, we create a temporary fix that can be fine-tuned or reversed, much like editing a draft rather than permanently altering the original manuscript. This approach introduces safer therapies with a reduced likelihood of unintended consequences associated with permanent modifications.

As this non-viral symphony continues to evolve, it promises to change the field of gene therapy. Each of these approaches offers unique advantages in modulating genetic expression and treating various diseases. While challenges remain, such as ensuring precise delivery and minimizing off-target effects, the growing repertoire of RNA-based therapies is composing a future where treatments are safer, more efficient, and more accessible than ever before.

Yet, the scientific community remains restless, constantly seeking new frontiers to explore. In this relentless pursuit of precision and control in genetic medicine, an earlier technology emerged, one that laid the foundation for targeted editing. As we continue to push the boundaries of what is possible in gene therapy, we are developing increasingly sophisticated methods for enhancing precision and control over interventions.

Zinc Finger Nuclease, or ZFN technology, allows for targeted modifications of DNA sequences and opens up new possibilities for correcting genetic defects. Zinc Finger Nucleases are engineered proteins that combine a DNA-binding zinc finger domain with a DNA-cleavage domain. This fusion allows it to target specific DNA sequences within complex genomes and create precise double-strand breaks at these sites. The zinc finger domains can be customized to recognize unique DNA sequences, enabling targeted gene editing with high specificity.

When they bind to their target DNA sequence, they induce double-strand breaks, which the cell's natural repair mechanisms then address. There are two primary pathways for repairing these breaks: non-homologous end joining and homologous recombination, also known as homology-directed repair. Non-homologous end joining often results in small insertions or deletions, which can disrupt gene function. In contrast, homology-directed repair can be used to introduce precise genetic changes using a donor DNA template.

The precision of these offers significant advantages for gene therapy. By targeting specific genes, zinc finger nucleases can potentially correct mutations responsible for genetic disorders such as hemophilia and Huntington's disease. This targeted approach minimizes the risks associated with traditional therapy methods that rely on viral vectors for random gene insertion.

These have been instrumental in creating animal models for human diseases. For instance, we have used zinc finger nucleases to induce specific mutations in zebrafish embryos, which serve as models for studying vascular diseases and other conditions. These models provide valuable insights into disease mechanisms and help develop new therapeutic strategies. Despite their potential, no zinc finger nuclease-based therapies have yet received full regulatory approval for widespread use as of 2025.

However, clinical trials are ongoing to assess the safety and efficacy of zinc finger nuclease-mediated therapies for conditions like HIV/AIDS and glioblastoma. Also, these have been considered and studied for use on hemophilia B, a blood clotting disorder caused by a deficiency in factor IX protein. They used zinc finger nucleases to insert a functional copy of the factor IX gene into liver cells. The liver is the body's primary site for factor IX production, so this approach aims to restore the body's ability to produce the crucial clotting factor.

While zinc finger nucleases offer remarkable precision, challenges remain in ensuring their safety and minimizing off-target effects. Unintended genetic modifications could have serious consequences, particularly in human applications. Moreover, the development of these requires time-consuming optimization processes to achieve the desired specificity and efficiency.

Transcription Activator-Like Effector Nucleases, or TALENs, expanded the gene-editing toolkit, offering a level of precision that was both awe-inspiring and transformative. Imagine the feeling of a key sliding effortlessly into a lock, each groove perfectly aligned. This is how TALENs interact with DNA, their protein fingers delicately tracing the contours of the genetic code.

TALENs are composed of two main components: a DNA-binding domain and a DNA-cleavage domain. TALENs are proteins that naturally bind to specific DNA sequences, and each repeat within these proteins corresponds to a single nucleotide in the target DNA sequence. This simple one-to-one correspondence allows us to design arrays that can bind to virtually any desired DNA sequence with high specificity.

Once bound to their target, they induce double-strand breaks in the DNA. This moment of controlled chaos within the cell is where the true magic happens. The cell's natural repair mechanisms, such as non-homologous end joining or homology-directed repair, kick into action to mend these breaks. This opens a window of opportunity to rewrite genetic stories, correcting mutations or introducing new genetic material.

This molecular sleight of hand is particularly poignant in the battle against cystic fibrosis. This relentless genetic foe turns the simple act of breathing into a daily struggle due to thick, suffocating mucus that clogs the lungs and obstructs the pancreas. Cystic fibrosis, often referred to as CF, is a disorder caused by mutations in the CFTR gene. It produces thick, suffocating mucus that can clog the lungs and obstruct the pancreas. By designing TALENs to target and repair these mutations specifically, the goal is to restore normal function to the CFTR gene, thereby alleviating symptoms and improving the quality of life for those affected.

Beyond cystic fibrosis, TALENs hold potential in treating hemoglobinopathies such as sickle cell disease and beta-thalassemia. These blood disorders result from mutations affecting hemoglobin production, leading to severe health complications. This hemoglobin is the vital protein in red blood cells that carries oxygen throughout the body. TALENs can be used to correct these mutations directly or reactivate fetal hemoglobin production, which can compensate for defective adult hemoglobin. This strategy offers hope for a long-term solution for patients suffering from these debilitating conditions.

The versatility of TALENs extends beyond human medicine into agriculture and biotechnology. They have been used to engineer disease-resistant crops, improve the nutritional qualities of food plants, and even create organisms that produce biofuel. In research settings, they facilitate precise genome modifications in various model organisms, advancing our understanding of genetics and opening new avenues.

Gene therapy is not just about molecules, enzymes, or cutting-edge tools—it's about people. Behind every breakthrough is a patient whose life hangs in the balance, a family searching for answers, and a story that reminds us why this work is so important. The promise of gene therapy comes alive when we move from the laboratory to the bedside, where science meets humanity.

CHAPTER 5

Triumphs and Tragedies

U p until now, we've explored the intricate world of DNA, genes, and gene therapies, delving into how we can understand and visualize them, as well as their direct impacts on medicine. Having gained this foundational understanding, we are ready to pivot towards the real-life implications of these advances. Let's delve into true personal stories that highlight the successes and challenges of gene therapies.

In the soft glow of a summer afternoon, a young boy's laughter echoes across a sun-dappled playground. His tiny feet kick up woodchips as he races towards the slide, his eyes bright with excitement. To the casual observer, he's just another carefree child reveling in the simple joys of childhood. But for those who know his story, every step, every giggle, every scraped knee is nothing short of miraculous.

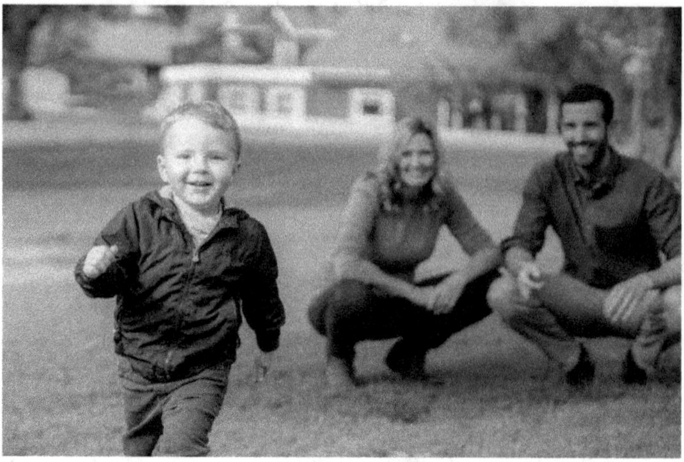

Figure 45. *Fitz Kettler and Family. Rady Children's Institute for Genomic Medicine.*

This is Fitz Kettler.

Rewind the clock to June 2019, and you'll find a very different scene. In the sterile confines of a neonatal intensive care unit, newborn Fitz lay in an incubator, his tiny body already engaged in a life-or-death struggle. The air was thick with the hum of medical equipment and the palpable anxiety of his parents.

The Kettlers' journey to parenthood had been a long one. When Fitz finally arrived, he seemed perfect – ten fingers and ten toes. But beneath his seemingly healthy exterior, a genetic time bomb was ticking. It was a routine newborn screening test that first raised the alarm.

Within days, advanced genetic sequencing confirmed the devastating diagnosis: Artemis-SCID, a rare and often fatal form of severe combined immunodeficiency. Fitz's body could not produce functioning immune cells, leaving him defenseless against even the most mundane infections.

In an instant, the Kettlers' world shrank to the confines of an isolation room at Rady Children's Hospital in San Diego. He had a rare and often fatal form of SCID, commonly known as "bubble boy disease." Without a functioning immune system, even minor infections could be life-threatening.

Doctors delivered the grim prognosis with gentle voices and averted eyes – without intervention, Fitz was unlikely to see his first birthday. Thanks to the early detection afforded by newborn screening, Fitz was a candidate for an experimental treatment. At just two months old, weighing no more than a small sack of flour, Fitz was whisked away to receive treatment.

At just two months old, Fitz underwent gene therapy at the University of California's Benioff Children's Hospital. His own stem cells were harvested, and a healthy copy of the gene responsible for his disease was given. In a 15-minute infusion, these modified cells were returned to Fitz's body, where they began producing healthy new immune cells. As the modified cells dripped into his tiny veins, the Kettlers could only wait and hope, their dreams for their son's future hanging by a thread as delicate as DNA.

Fast forward to today, in the warm glow of a sunny afternoon, Fitz Kettler races across the playground, his laughter mingling with the sounds of other children at play. He attends preschool, builds towering Lego structures, and, yes, occasionally succumbs to the sniffles – each mundane illness a quiet celebration of his functioning immune system. To an observer, he's just like any other preschooler, full of energy and life. But to his parents, every giggle and tumble is a testament to the miracles of modern medicine.

To see this energetic preschooler today, you'd never guess the harrowing journey that brought him here. Without early detection,

Fitz's condition might have gone unnoticed until a life-threatening infection struck. Today, four-year-old Fitz Kettler stands on his stepstool at the kitchen counter, eagerly helping his mom stir cupcake batter. His infectious giggles fill the room as he sneaks a taste of the sweet batter.

He is an active, healthy preschooler with a robust immune system. For the Kettlers, watching their son thrive is a daily reminder of how newborn screening and gene therapy saved his life. Fitz's experience is not unique.

~●

For Opal, silence had always been her constant companion. Opal was born with a genetic condition that left her completely deaf. As a result, she uniquely experienced the world, navigating through a universe devoid of sound. Her parents' soothing words were gentle vibrations against her skin, and the joyful laughter of others unfolded like a silent movie.

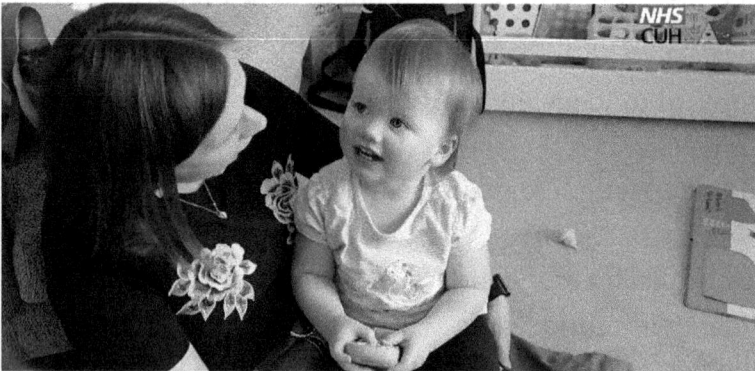

Figure 46. Baby Opal and Her Mother Jo. Cambridge University Hospitals NHS Foundation Trust

Opal's parents, Jo and James Sandy, were determined to find a solution to their daughter's condition. They spared no effort in seeking expert guidance and meticulously exploring every available treatment option. Traditional treatments presented limited alternatives, with the potential benefit of cochlear implants being the primary option. However, they recognized that these devices didn't fully replicate natural hearing experiences.

Then came a new possibility in the form of gene therapy. This approach promised to address the root cause of Opal's deafness by repairing the defect. The Sandys were torn between lingering skepticism and a growing sense of excitement as they dared to dream that this treatment might be the breakthrough they desperately sought.

To understand the potential of gene therapy for hearing loss, it's essential to grasp the basics of how hearing works and what goes wrong with genetic deafness. The journey of sound perception begins in the cochlea, a delicate, spiral-shaped structure within the inner ear housing specialized hair cells. These cells convert sound vibrations into electrical signals and transmit them to the brain. However, mutations can disrupt this intricate process, leading to hearing loss or deafness.

In Opal's case, the culprit was a mutation in the Otoferlin gene. This specific gene plays a crucial role in producing the otoferlin protein, which is essential for enabling communication between the cells of the inner ear and the nerve fibers responsible for hearing. When the otoferlin protein is not functioning correctly, the transmission of sound signals is significantly impaired.

The Sandys considered enrolling Opal in the CHORD trial, an international phase 1/2 clinical study. This decision meant that

Opal would participate in a research study to assess the safety and effectiveness of a new treatment. This trial focuses on exploring the use of gene therapy to treat children with severe hearing loss caused by specific gene mutations. For families like the Sandys, grappling with similar medical challenges, this trial provided a ray of optimism amidst an otherwise overwhelming scenario.

As a precaution against potential adverse effects, a small dose of gene therapy was carefully and precisely applied to one of Opal's ears. The treatment process included a precise injection into the cochlea while Opal was under general anesthesia. Specially designed vectors targeted the cochlea's inner hair cells, facilitating the release of the correct otoferlin gene. This allowed for the production of the essential protein needed for the treatment.

The weeks following the treatment were filled with anxious anticipation. Then, one day, the deafening silence was shattered as Opal heard her parents clapping for the first time. "When Opal could hear us clapping unaided, it was mind-blowing," Jo Sandy recalls. "We were so happy when the clinical team confirmed at 24 weeks that her hearing was also picking up softer sounds and speech."

While the initial results showed promise, it's essential to acknowledge the study's limitations. The trial is still in its early stages, and long-term data on the treatment's durability and potential side effects are not yet available. It's worth noting that gene therapy carries inherent risks, including immune responses and unforeseen complications.

Dr. Richard Brown, Consultant Paediatrician at Cambridge University Hospital and Investigator on the CHORD trial, emphasizes the need for caution. "It is likely that in the long run, such treatments require less follow-up, so they may prove to be an attractive option, including within the developing world. Follow-up appointments have shown effective results with no adverse reactions, and it is exciting to see the results to date."

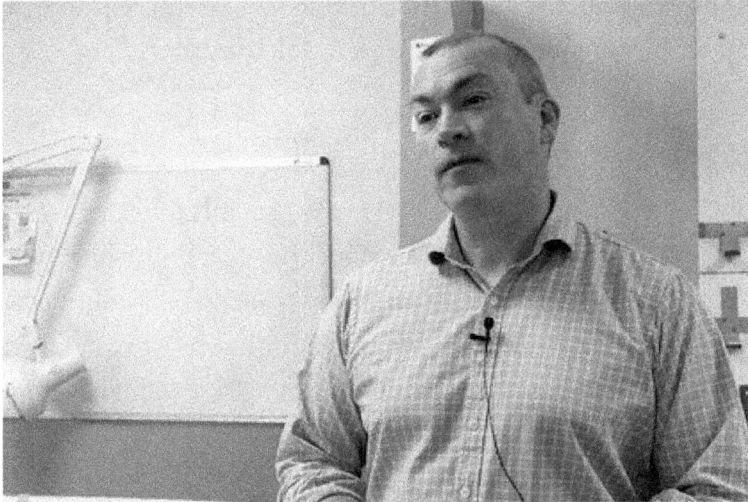

Figure 47. *Richard Brown. Cambridge University Hospitals NHS Foundation Trust*

The success of Opal's gene therapy provides a promising glimpse into the future of treating genetic hearing loss. Unlike traditional cochlear implants, this therapy can be a transformative option for individuals with otoferlin mutations, offering a more organic and natural approach to addressing their hearing challenges.

However, the road ahead is challenging. High treatment costs, ethical considerations, and potential long-term effects must be carefully navigated. Extensive research and clinical trials are necessary to ensure the safety and efficacy of these therapies. Regulatory hurdles and funding are critical factors in bringing these treatments from the lab to the clinic.

Opal's story underscores the transformative potential of gene therapy, not just for those with genetic deafness but for countless other conditions. Dr. Richard Brown captures the essence of this new era. "The development of genomic medicine and alternative treatments is vital for patients worldwide and increasingly offers hope to children with previously incurable disorders."

~❧

But not every tale is one of victory. Recall the story of Jesse Gelsinger. These stories serve as a stark contrast. Some families have faced the harsh realities of gene therapy gone awry—patients whose bodies rejected treatments or whose conditions worsened despite the promise of cutting-edge science. These stories serve as poignant reminders that setbacks and heartache often accompany progress.

A potential new medical era was brewing in the sterile corridors of Hôpital Necker-Enfants Malades in Paris. It was 2000, and the air buzzed with an electric mix of hope. Dr. Alain Fischer, a pediatric immunologist with kind eyes and a determined set to his jaw, stood at the precipice of history. In his hands, he held not just a syringe but the dreams of countless families and the future of medicine itself.

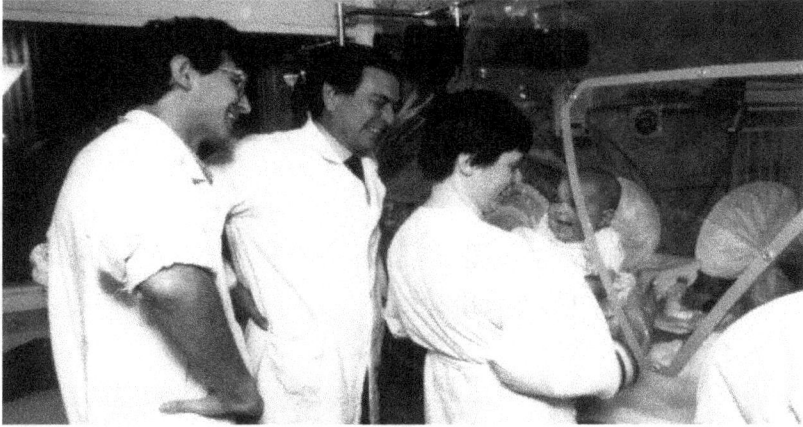

Figure 48. Alain Fischer and Claude Griscelli. Alain Fischer and Radio France

Severe combined immunodeficiency or SCID, as we've seen before, had long been a death sentence. Children born with this rare genetic disorder lacked the basic immune defenses to fight off even the most mundane infections. Their world was one of isolation, sterile rooms, and the constant hum of air filters. Parents could only touch their children through thick plastic gloves, their love separated by an impenetrable barrier.

At just 8 months old, one such child peered out from behind a plastic shield, never having felt the touch of his mother's skin or the warmth of a real hug. His parents had all but given up hope until they heard about Dr. Fischer's trial. It was like being offered a ticket to the moon; it was impossible, yet they desperately wanted to believe.

The trial began with a mix of fanfare and cautious optimism. One by one, children receive the modified virus carrying the healthy gene their bodies so desperately need. The world held its breath, waiting. And then, like flowers blooming after a long winter, the children's immune systems flourished.

The 8-month-old boy's blood tests showed a steady climb in T-cell counts. For the first time, he fought off a common cold without complication. The day he left the sterile room, taking his first steps into the bustling hospital corridor, there wasn't a dry eye. They had done it. They had given these children a future.

For three glorious years, the trial's success seemed unassailable. The children thrived. They attended school, made friends, and experienced the simple joys that had once been forbidden: a trip to the park, a family vacation, a birthday party with other kids. But in the quiet of a late-night lab, a researcher noticed something alarming in a routine blood test. They checked and rechecked the results, praying it was a mistake.

The news hit like a thunderbolt. One of the trial's first patients had developed leukemia. The very treatment that had saved him was now threatening his life in a cruel twist of cellular fate. The treatment used a modified virus, a retroviral vector. This vector was designed to sneak a healthy copy of the defective gene into the patient's DNA.

The complication arose from insertional mutagenesis. The viral vector, carrying its payload of therapeutic genes, inserted itself randomly into the patients' chromosomes. This randomness was the treatment's Achilles' heel.

Sometimes, the vector accidentally lands near genes that control cell growth and division, known as proto-oncogenes. The vector carried a powerful promoter sequence intended to boost the expression of the therapeutic gene. However, this promoter could also activate nearby genes it was never meant to influence.

In the French trials, the vector was inserted near a gene called LMO-2, which is involved in the development of childhood cancers. The vector's promoter inadvertently activated this gene, leading to uncontrolled T-cell growth. The activation of LMO-2 and possibly other growth-control genes caused specific T cells to proliferate unchecked, leading to a leukemia-like condition. It was a direct, though unintended, consequence of the gene therapy—a cruel twist of cellular fate.

As more cases emerged, the triumph turned to tragedy. Five of 20 patients treated in similar trials in France and the UK developed leukemia. While this percentage is significant and alarming, it also means that the majority of patients did not experience this severe side effect. The gene therapy community, once riding high on success, now found itself in free fall. Emergency meetings were called, trials were halted, and the promise of a new medical frontier seemed to crumble.

The following years were a crucible of soul-searching, rigorous research, and painstaking improvements. The scientific community, humbled but not defeated, worked tirelessly to understand what had happened and how to prevent it. For families impacted by the therapies, the journey was complex. Many don't regret their choice as they now watch their children play in the backyard – a sight they once thought impossible. But they live with the fear, always, that something may change or cancer may be on the horizon.

The juxtaposition of gene therapy's hopeful journey and the sobering reality of the trial highlights the path of progress. The landscape of gene therapy has been marred by setbacks, particularly in light of the unfortunate outcomes of the SCID trials. The community, however, did not falter in its pursuit of innovation and healing.

In this evolving narrative of resilience and progress, we find the inspiring story of Noa Greenwood. Lee and Lori Greenwood, a typical Boston couple, had dreams for their daughter, Noa. As new parents, they were attentive to every detail of her development.

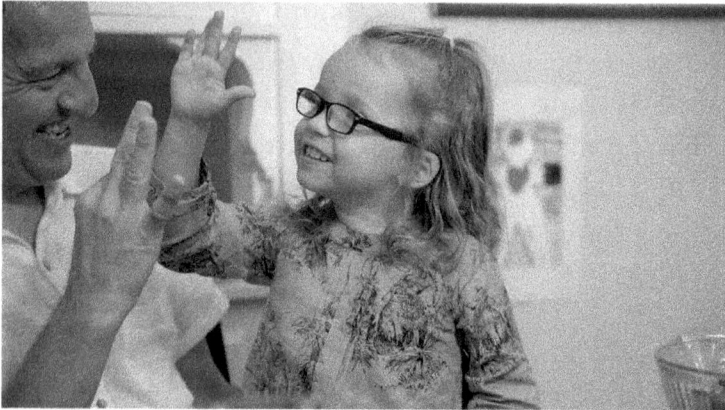

Figure 49. Noa and Lee Greenwood. Bryan Goodchild for UMass Chan Medical School

However, when they noticed unusual signs around eight weeks old, excessive crying and difficulty gaining weight, their world began to unravel. What followed was a harrowing journey filled with uncertainty and fear, but also a shining example of how the lessons learned from past trials can lead to new avenues of hope and potential healing for conditions like Canavan disease.

Their world changed when, at just 11 months old, Noa was diagnosed with Canavan disease. This rare, devastating genetic disorder affects the central nervous system, muscles, and eyes. The news hit them like thunderclaps, shattering their hopes and dreams for their little girl. As symptoms emerged, muscle weakness and loss of head control, the Greenwood family found themselves on an emotional rollercoaster, grappling with despair while searching for answers.

But amid the darkness, a glimmer of hope appeared. When they learned about a clinical trial for Canavan disease at Massachusetts General Hospital, just 30 minutes from their home, they felt the stirrings of possibility. This trial represented a treatment and a chance to reclaim Noa's future.

The medical trial CANaspire, led by Dr. Florian Eichler at Mass General Hospital, aimed to address the underlying cause of Canavan disease, which occurs when a gene called ASPA doesn't work correctly. It makes an enzyme that breaks down a substance in the brain. When it builds up, it can interfere with the brain's normal development, particularly affecting the protective coating around nerve cells called myelin.

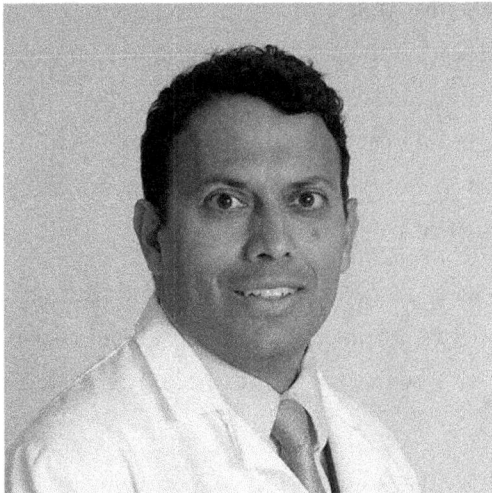

Figure 50. Florian Eichler. Massachusetts General Hospital

The Greenwoods were cautiously optimistic when Noa was declared eligible for the trial. In June 2022, at 22 months, Noa became the third child to receive a dose of this gene therapy. For the family, the stakes couldn't have been higher. The treatment held hope, yet the air was thick with uncertainty. *Would this be the solution they've been hoping for, the awaited answer to their prayers?*

The day Noa received her first dose of gene therapy, the room buzzed with nervous excitement. Lee and Lori stood by, and an electric energy filled the room. Their hearts raced, and their minds swirled with questions and what-ifs. As the treatment was administered, time seemed to stand still, a singular moment suspended in the air. What followed was a period of intense waiting, monitoring every small change and holding on with each passing moment.

In the following months, the Greenwoods celebrated numerous small yet significant achievements. Noa's development gradually improved. She began to show signs of what any parent would cherish: sitting up in her booster seat, feeding herself snacks, and joyfully babbling to her parents. For Lee and Lori, these moments were nothing short of miraculous.

Dr. Elisabet Mandon, a member of the gene therapy research team, couldn't conceal her amazement. "I can't believe it. I'm shocked. Looking at her, she is not a 2-year-old patient with Canavan," she remarked.

Noa's progress blended joy, relief, and ongoing uncertainty for the Greenwood family. Every milestone was celebrated, but the weight of being pioneers in this experimental therapy was never far from their minds.

Noa's future is uncertain as gene therapy is still in the early investigational stages. However, the progress she has made provides for a better tomorrow, not only for Noa but also for many others dealing with genetic disorders. Alongside Noa's journey, another bolt of lightning struck.

Marie-Chantal's story begins with the heartrending moments of her childhood as a toddler who couldn't play in the snow because the cold could trigger a debilitating pain episode. This pain, known as a pain crisis, was a constant shadow in her life. It wasn't just the physical agony; it was the emotional toll of feeling different and restricted. For many, like Marie-Chantal, sickle cell disease is not just a medical condition; it's a relentless adversary that affects every aspect of life.

As she entered her teenage years, the frequency and intensity of her pain crises began to escalate. The pain became increasingly severe, with over-the-counter medications providing little relief, necessitating frequent hospital admissions for more potent interventions. Dr. Alexis Thompson, Chief of the Division of Hematology at Children's Hospital of Philadelphia, sheds light on the burden of this disease, saying, "This pain for some is almost indescribable. It causes an extraordinary burden to the individual and their families, requiring emergency room visits or hospitalizations."

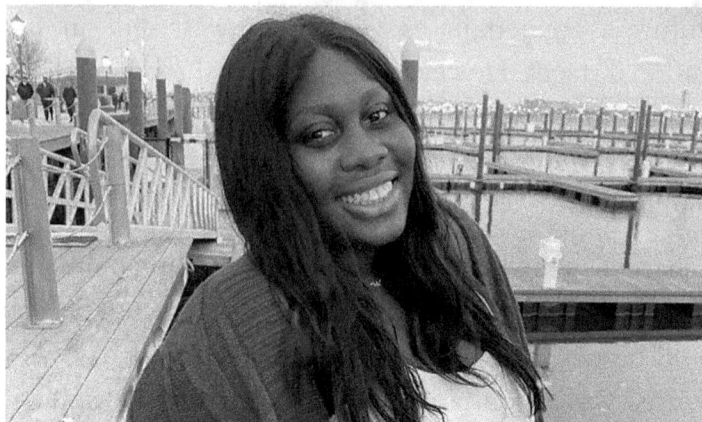

Figure 51. Marie-Chantal. The Children's Hospital of Philadelphia

A single gene mutation causes sickle cell disease. It predominantly affects people of African and Middle Eastern descent. This mutation leads to the production of abnormal hemoglobin, which distorts red blood cells into a rigid, sticky, crescent shape. These misshapen cells can obstruct blood flow, causing severe pain and organ damage.

Recently, the effectiveness of medications in maintaining the round shape of red blood cells has been limited. The primary treatment for sickle cell disease has been a bone marrow transplant from a compatible sibling donor, which has made it inaccessible to many individuals. Marie's brother also carried the sickle cell trait and, therefore, turned out to be an unsuitable match for donation.

Marie's life underwent a significant transformation shortly before her 21st birthday. She decided to take part in a clinical trial for gene therapy. This treatment, called CASGEVY, received FDA approval on December 8, 2023. It harnesses CRISPR technology to correct the genetic mutation responsible for sickle cell disease precisely.

"More than 90% of individuals are pain-free following gene therapy. That's an extraordinary accomplishment," says Dr. Alexis Thompson, who was involved in the early development of this therapy. The process involves extracting bone marrow stem cells from the patient, editing them in a lab to produce normal hemoglobin, and then reinfusing them after a round of chemotherapy. This procedure, akin to a bone marrow transplant, is safer as it eliminates the need for a donor and reduces the risk of rejection.

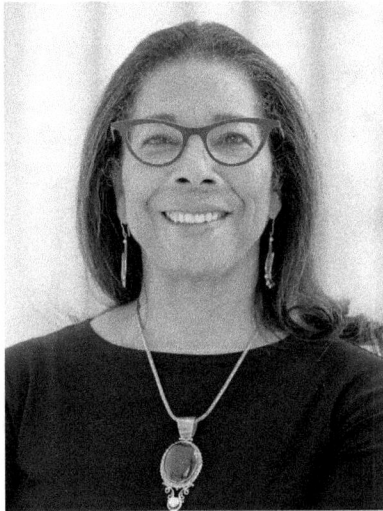

Figure 52. Alexis A. Thompson. The Children's Hospital of Philadelphia

Marie is now pain-free. For her, the transformation is profound. More importantly, she envisions a future she once thought impossible. "The life expectancy for someone with sickle cell disease is usually up to the 50s. Now, I can see myself living into my 80s or 90s. I can imagine the life I'll have, the family I'll build, and my future. I'm incredibly excited," she says.

Marie-Chantal's story is a powerful testament to the potential of gene therapy to transform lives. The journey of those undergoing treatment, filled with challenges and triumphs, underscores the importance of continued research and innovation in this field. Yet, as science races forward, each breakthrough also brings new questions—about what we can know, what we should change, and how far we are willing to go in rewriting the scripts written in our genes. It is at this crossroads of hope and uncertainty that the next chapter begins.

CHAPTER 6

Pandora's Box: The Promise and Perils of Genetic Knowledge

In a quiet hospital nursery, a nurse gently lifts a newborn's tiny foot. With practiced precision, she pricks the heel, collecting a few drops of blood on a special card. This simple act, performed countless times each day across the nation, has become a silent guardian of our most vulnerable. By 2024, this heel prick test had become as routine as a lullaby in 48 states and Washington, D.C., safeguarding an astounding 99% of newborns in the United States.

Those few crimson drops, no larger than a teardrop, now stand as a formidable frontline defense against the cruel randomness of genetic disorders. The significance of this test becomes strikingly clear when seen through the eyes of families whose lives it has changed forever.

The Villarreals watched with a mix of joy and trepidation, marveling at Evelyn's delicate fingers and perfect pink toes, counting each tiny breath, and imagining the bright future ahead of her, as the nurse prepared their daughter, Evelyn, for the routine newborn screening. Like all new parents, they dreamed of first words, first steps, and countless milestones yet to come. But *unlike* most families, the Villarreals were about to face an invisible threat—one that could have stolen Evelyn's future before it had even begun.

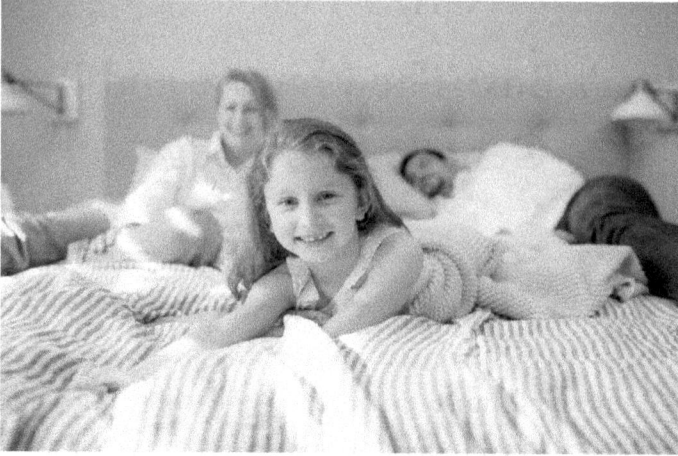

Figure 53. *Evelyn and her parents, Milan & Elena. Villarreal family & CDC*

Just days later, the hospital room that had been filled with Evelyn's soft coos and her parents' whispered dreams now felt unbearably heavy with silence. Milan and Elena sat with their hands clasped tightly. The doctor entered with a grave expression that spoke volumes before he uttered a single word.

The routine heel prick test, a simple procedure they had barely given a second thought to, had revealed a devastating truth: their precious Evelyn had spinal muscular atrophy or SMA. The words fell like hammer blows, each syllable shattering their dreams for their daughter's future.

SMA was a diagnosis that once meant certain tragedy; a life marked by increasing frailty and loss. At that moment, it felt as if the very air had been sucked from the room, leaving them gasping for breath and grasping for hope. Milan and Elena could almost see the milestones they had envisioned for Evelyn slipping away: her first laugh, her first steps, her first day at school. All of it now seemed impossibly out of reach.

In years past, this diagnosis would have been a death sentence. But Evelyn was born into a new era. One where science and medicine had begun rewriting fate's cruelest scripts. Within weeks of her diagnosis, Evelyn was enrolled in a gene therapy trial in Ohio.

As the doctors prepared to administer the therapy, the air in the room grew thick with anticipation. This wasn't just about inserting a functional copy of the SMN1 gene into Evelyn's tiny body—it was about rewriting her genetics. Every beep of the medical equipment and every twitch of Evelyn's little fingers seemed loaded with significance.

Days turned into weeks, weeks into months. Each day brought new anxieties and new hopes. *Would Evelyn lift her head today? Would she grasp a toy?*

Each milestone, no matter how small, became a cause for celebration. It was a potential sign that the treatment was working its microscopic magic. The Villarreal home began to fill with sounds they had once feared they might never hear: Evelyn's laughter, her first words, the pitter-patter of unsteady feet.

Today, Evelyn is a lively child, her laughter echoing through the Villarreal home. Her parents watch in awe as she reaches developmental milestones they once feared she might never achieve. Each wobbly step and each babbled word is a testament to the power of genetic screening and the wonders of modern medicine.

The concept of genetic screening has exploded beyond its humble beginnings in newborn care and stands to redefine healthcare as we know it. Universal screening, once a pipe dream, now looms on the horizon. This ambitious vision seeks to democratize genetic insight, offering every individual, regardless of age or current health status, a chance to decode their DNA's secrets.

Imagine a sterile, white-walled room, where a young woman, let's call her Sarah, is sitting perched on the edge of a cold metal chair. Her heart pounds a staccato rhythm against her ribs. The antiseptic smell burns her nostrils, a stark reminder of why she's here.

This isn't the routine heel prick of a newborn, a test performed without conscious choice. No, Sarah has made this decision, driven by a potent cocktail of fear and dreams, to peer into the very core of her genetic makeup.

The weight of her mother's recent breast cancer diagnosis hangs heavy in the air, as tangible as the vial of blood now cradled in the lab technician's gloved hands. Sarah's eyes follow the vial, that crimson liquid holding the blueprint of her existence, as it's whisked away for analysis.

Days pass, and Sarah's anxiety grows. She imagines her genes unraveling like a thread; each decoded base pair is another piece of her genetic puzzle. Finally, the day arrives. Sarah sits in the genetic counselor's office, her palms slick with sweat as she awaits her results. As she waits, she can't help but think about her younger sister and teenage niece.

Would her decision to get tested also impact their lives?

The counselor's face is a mask of professional neutrality as she begins to speak. "Your test results show a mutation in the BRCA1 gene," the counselor explains gently. "This increases your risk of developing breast and ovarian cancer."

The words hit Sarah like a physical blow. Her heart races as the implications sink in. Upon learning of her BRCA1 mutation, Sarah's face was a canvas of emotions: fear, shock, and then, gradually, steely determination.

Her fingers, adorned with perfectly manicured nails, gripped the armrests of the chair as she absorbed the news. She thinks of her sister again, her teenage niece. *Should she tell them? Do they have a right to know? Do they have a right not to know?*

As if flipping a switch, Sarah's posture had changed. Her spine straightened, her chin lifted, and a fire ignited in her eyes. *"Okay,"* she had said, her voice steady despite the slight tremor in her hands, *"what do we do now?"*

From that moment, Sarah embarked on a journey of proactive health management. Her genetic information had become a roadmap, each data point a signpost guiding her toward a future where she felt in control. Sarah's story is just one of countless stories playing out across the globe.

Recall Amy, the geneticist we met at the beginning of this book, sitting in her office after hours. The soft glow of her computer screen illuminates her face, casting shadows that seem to dance with the weight of her knowledge. Her finger hovers over the mouse, trembling slightly as she contemplates whether she wants to complete testing and receive her genetic test results.

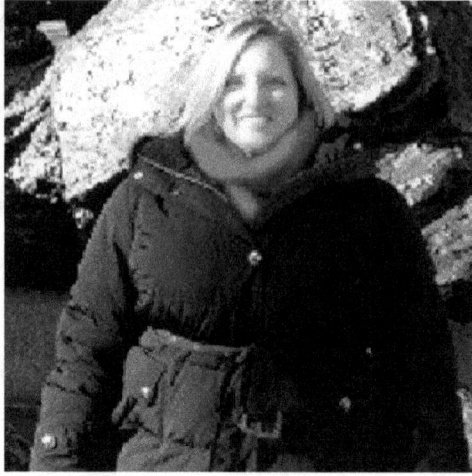

Figure 54. Amy. CDC

The irony isn't lost on her - she's guided countless others through this very moment, yet here she is, paralyzed by the prospect of her genetic reckoning. The hesitation that gripped her was visceral, a physical force that seemed to root her to her chair. It resonated so deeply that she could almost hear the echoes of her patients' voices, their fears and hopes mingling with her own in a cacophony of uncertainty.

For years, she had been the calm voice of reason, the steady hand guiding others through the stormy seas of genetic uncertainty. Now, she found herself adrift, clinging to the wreckage of her professional detachment as the waves of personal fear threatened to pull her under.

Her family history loomed large in her mind. Five relatives claimed by cancer's merciless grip, three before they even saw their 40th birthday. The specter of Lynch Syndrome, that cruel legacy, seemed to hover in the room, its cold fingers reaching for her.

To undergo screening was to change the narrative of her life, to step from the realm of blissful uncertainty into stark, genetic reality. Despite her profound understanding of the significance of refusing testing, Amy decided not to go forward with the screening, choosing the comfort of *not knowing*.

Three days after her 47th birthday, Amy's world shifted. What she had dismissed as a minor discomfort was a harbinger of devastating news. The doctor's words came down with crushing weight: *"Stage 3 colorectal cancer."*

"I rationalized that it couldn't happen to me," Amy whispered, the words catching in her throat. Even as they left her lips, she recognized the fallacy of her thinking. A bitter laugh escaped her – *how many times had she gently corrected this very notion in her patients?*

The science was clear, brutally so. It didn't discriminate. It didn't care about degrees or expertise. It was a lottery, and her ticket had been punched the moment she was conceived.

In the whirlwind of tests, consultations, and sleepless nights, the test she had avoided became an unavoidable reality. The results confirmed what she had feared all along: she carried the MSH2 mutation, the genetic signature of the disease that had haunted her family for generations.

As Amy navigated the grueling path of cancer treatment, she found herself on a parallel journey of self-discovery and purpose. The geneticist became the patient, and the advisor is now the advocate. She channeled her fear and pain into a fierce determination to prevent others from facing the same ordeal.

Social media became her pulpit, and her story was a rallying cry for awareness of Lynch Syndrome. She urged others to take preventative measures, and her professional knowledge became a lifeline for her own family. *Every post, every share, every conversation* became a small victory in her war against the disease that had ambushed her.

In the quiet moments between treatments, Amy often reflected on that night in her office when fear had held her back from the knowledge that might have changed everything. Now, she understood that the true power of genetic information lies not in knowing, but in the actions we take because of it.

Amy knew all too well that the psychological impact of the knowledge could be as varied as the human genome itself. In her years as a geneticist, she had witnessed the full spectrum of human reactions to this most intimate revelation. Now, as she lay in her bed, the weight of her genetic reality pressing down on her, these memories came flooding back with vivid intensity.

Some, like Sarah, find empowerment in understanding their risks. But then there are others. For example, Mark is a 48-year-old active father of two, for whom genetic knowledge casts a long, dark shadow over every aspect of life.

He could be found sitting at his kitchen table, the cheerful yellow walls a stark contrast to the gloom that enveloped him. His hands wrapped around a mug of coffee gone cold, eyes distant and haunted. The steam had dissipated, like the warmth that once filled his eyes when he spoke of his children's future.

Now, those eyes were distant and haunted, focused on some point far beyond the present moment. The lines etched around them spoke not of laughter but of sleepless nights and constant worry. The kitchen clock ticked loudly in the silence, each second a reminder of the genetic time bomb ticking within him.

The gene associated with early-onset Alzheimer's disease that lurked in Mark's DNA had become an invisible, ever-present companion. It whispered doubts into his ear with every forgotten name, every misplaced set of keys. This morning, a forgotten dentist appointment sent his heart racing, his palms sweating as he fumbled to reschedule. Every time he forgets something, he wonders: *Is this it? Has it started?*

The weight of Mark's anxiety permeated his every waking moment, a heavy blanket that smothered joy and amplified fear. Simple acts of forgetfulness that were once brushed off as normal now took on ominous significance. He found himself pausing mid-sentence, a flicker of panic crossing his face as he struggled to recall a common word.

Was this just a normal lapse or the first sign of the disease that had become his constant dread?

Desperate to cling to every memory fragment, Mark had become obsessive in his quest for order and recall. His once-steady hands now shook slightly as he scribbled reminders on every available surface. Post-it notes covered his refrigerator, a kaleidoscope of yellow, pink, and blue squares bearing crucial information. They also framed his computer screen, and even the bathroom mirror wasn't spared, its reflective surface partially obscured by reminders of appointments, birthdays, and daily tasks.

In the living room, a wall calendar hung, each day's square crammed with tiny, careful handwriting. Mark's eyes darted to it frequently, checking and rechecking upcoming events. On the kitchen counter, a series of pill organizers stood in neat rows, a physical manifestation of his determination to stay healthy, to fight against the genetic hand he'd been dealt.

The future Mark had once looked forward to with excitement, watching his children grow and planning for retirement with his wife, now loomed before him like a dark, uncertain void. Each milestone was overshadowed by the question: *Will I still be myself when that day comes?*

He looked at the refrigerator, dotted with his children's artwork and school photos, and felt a sense of fear.

Would he recognize these precious faces in five years? Ten?

The contrast is stark - Sarah's empowerment against Mark's despair - yet both are valid, deeply human responses to the weight of the information. Genetic screening has immense potential benefits despite these challenges, risks, and anxieties. Early detection can lead to life-saving interventions, help families make informed decisions about future pregnancies, and even guide more personalized and effective care. The knowledge we've gained from understanding DNA is not just a tool for prediction; it's becoming a powerful instrument for prevention and treatment.

~~❧~~

As we navigate this new world of genetic discovery, we must also reflect on the nonmedical implications of sequencing and its familial nature. One case in particular stands out above all others and illustrates the profound impacts of genetic testing beyond individual health: it highlights that information does not exist in a vacuum; its implications extend far beyond the individual.

In a hushed courtroom in New South Wales, Australia, Kathleen Folbigg sat motionless, her face a mosaic of emotions: hope, fear, exhaustion. The air was thick with anticipation, the silence broken only by the faint shuffle of papers and the rhythmic ticking of the clock. For 20 years, Kathleen had lived under the weight of a damning narrative: she was "Australia's worst mother," convicted of killing her four children. But today, as she waited for the judge's decision, science had finally given her a voice.

It began in the 1980s when Folbigg's four children, Caleb, Patrick, Sarah, and Laura, died suddenly and inexplicably. They were all so young, ranging from just 19 days to 19 months old. Each death was initially attributed to natural causes: sudden infant death syndrome (SIDS) or other unexplained factors.

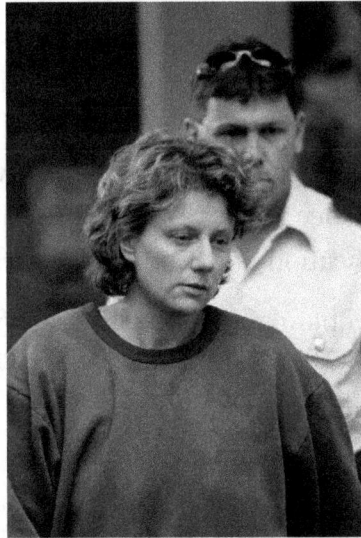

Figure 55. Kathleen Folbigg. Anita Jones/Fairfax Media & Nature

But as the years passed and the losses accumulated, suspicion began to mount. The rarity of multiple SIDS deaths in a single family led authorities to question whether something more sinister was at play. Whispers of foul play grew louder.

Kathleen's troubled past only fueled these suspicions. Her father had murdered her mother when Kathleen was just 18 months old, and prosecutors painted her as a woman shaped by violence—a mother who had turned that violence inward on her own children. The turning point came when Kathleen's husband discovered her personal diaries and handed them over to the police.

In them were entries that prosecutors interpreted as confessions: expressions of guilt and anguish that they claimed revealed her culpability. To Kathleen, these were the words of a grieving mother consumed by self-doubt; to prosecutors, they were evidence of murder.

In 2003, despite no direct evidence linking her to the deaths, Kathleen was convicted of three counts of murder, one count of manslaughter, and one count of grievous bodily harm. She was sentenced to 40 years in prison. The sentence was later reduced to 30 on appeal. For two decades, she maintained her innocence while enduring public vilification and repeated legal defeats.

Everything began to change in 2018 when a group petitioned for a review of her case based on genetic evidence. They discovered that Folbigg's two daughters carried a rare mutation in the CALM2 gene, which can cause sudden cardiac death in infants and children. Later analysis revealed that her two sons carried mutations in the BSN gene, which is associated with lethal epileptic seizures.

These discoveries challenged the foundation of Folbigg's conviction. They offered a plausible, natural explanation for the tragic deaths of her children. This explanation had been impossible to uncover with the scientific tools available at the time of her trial.

As Folbigg sat in that courtroom in June 2023, awaiting the decision to rewrite her story, she embodied the profound impact that advances in genetic science can have on justice, truth, and individual lives. The judge's voice rang out, *"On the basis of the new scientific evidence, there is a reasonable doubt as to Ms. Folbigg's guilt."*

This revelation didn't just lead to Folbigg's pardon; it shattered the foundations of a two-decade-old narrative. It forced everyone present - from the judge to the spectators - to confront the power and responsibility of unraveling the secrets hidden in our genes. As Folbigg left the courtroom, free for the first time in 20 years, she stepped into a world forever changed by science.

While it brought freedom and vindication for Kathleen, it also forced society to confront uncomfortable truths about its rush to judgment and its failure to understand the complexities of science at the time of her trial. Her case became a stark reminder of how advances in research can rewrite not just individual lives but entire narratives.

The implications rippled far beyond Kathleen herself. Sequencing her genome had not only exonerated her but also rewritten her family's medical history. Her children's deaths were no longer inexplicable tragedies but part of a genetic legacy. A legacy that could potentially affect extended family members for generations to come.

While providing answers to long-standing questions, this legacy also opened up a Pandora's box of ethical and legal considerations. The power of genetic information to reshape narratives and impact lives across generations is a double-edged sword, as evidenced by the growing concerns surrounding law enforcement's use of databases.

The use of genetic information by law enforcement agencies has become increasingly prevalent, raising significant privacy concerns. Police are now turning to both public and private data sources, which contain vast amounts of gene information. This practice has led to the solving of cold cases. Still, it has also sparked debates about individual privacy rights and potential misuse.

One of the primary concerns is the lack of robust legal frameworks to govern law enforcement's use of genetic data. In some cases, police have obtained warrants to access entire databases, regardless of user consent. This broad access could potentially expose individuals who have voluntarily submitted their DNA and their relatives who may be unaware of their genetic information being indirectly accessible.

Several states have begun to address these concerns through legislation. For instance, Maryland has narrowed access to only those databases that explicitly inform consumers about potential law enforcement use. Utah has passed bipartisan legislation defining the circumstances under which law enforcement can request the use of genetic databases and limiting the types of charges and arrests that can be based on specific information.

The balance between its potential benefits for solving crimes and the need to protect individual privacy remains a critical issue. Lawmakers and policymakers face the challenge of creating regulations that allow for the responsible use of genetic information while safeguarding the rights and well-being of individuals and their families.

Effective regulation and oversight are essential to ensure that genetic technologies are used responsibly and ethically. Governments, scientific organizations, and professional bodies must work together to develop clear guidelines and standards for genetic testing, gene therapy, and other interventions. These regulations should address issues such as informed consent, data privacy, genetic discrimination, and the safety and efficacy of technologies.

~❦~

In the realm of genetic screening, there are profound questions about privacy and the potential for discrimination. The anxiety surrounding the potential for discrimination is not just a theoretical concern. For example, the dark shadow of eugenics looms large over the past, a chilling reminder of how genetic information can be weaponized against the vulnerable.

In the early 20th century, a pseudoscientific movement swept across the nation, disguised as an effort to "improve" humanity. This movement, fueled by racism and xenophobia, sought to sculpt the gene pool through forced sterilization and selective breeding. By 1931, 30 American states had enshrined eugenic ideologies into law, resulting in the forced sterilization of over 64,000 people, primarily targeting the poor, mentally ill, and people of color.

The impact of these laws varied by state. For example, North Carolina's program was particularly aggressive, allowing social workers to designate individuals for sterilization. Oklahoma sterilized 556 individuals, with 78% being female. The most significant era of eugenic sterilization in the United States spanned from 1907 to 1963. As recently as the 1970s, some populations of Americans were subjected to coerced sterilizations.

This dark chapter wasn't confined to the United States. Eugenics had become a global movement, gaining popular, elite, and governmental support in countries such as Germany, Great Britain, Italy, Mexico, and Canada. Proponents from various fields, including statisticians, economists, anthropologists, sociologists, geneticists, and public health officials, championed eugenic ideas through academic and popular literature.

The most notorious application of eugenics occurred in Nazi Germany from 1933 to 1945. The Nazi regime weaponized these ideas to "cleanse" German society of those deemed "unworthy of life." Their campaign of terror included the euthanasia of at least 70,000 adults and 5,200 children and the forced sterilization of over 400,000 individuals. This culminated in the Holocaust, targeting Jews, Sinti and Roma people, individuals with disabilities, and LGBTQ+ people.

This isn't ancient history. The echoes of this dark chapter reverberate today in our fears about genetic discrimination. When we worry about employers or insurers accessing our DNA, we're not being paranoid, as there *was* a time when genetic "fitness" determined who could work, marry, and have children.

More recent and contemporary concerns about discrimination echo these historical injustices. Take Terri Sergeant, for example. A driven and capable manager at a small insurance brokerage in North Carolina, Terri had built a promising career through hard work and dedication.

But her life unraveled after she was diagnosed with alpha-1 antitrypsin deficiency, a genetic condition that affects the lungs and liver. With medication, the condition was manageable. But her employer didn't see it that way. The diagnosis wasn't just a medical label; it became a scarlet letter. Shortly after her condition became known, Terri was fired.

The dismissal was more than just a professional blow—it was the first domino in a cascade of devastation. Without her job, she lost her health insurance, which had been her only way to afford the expensive medication to keep her condition under control. As her untreated symptoms worsened, so did her ability to find new work. Her once-bright future dimmed, replaced by mounting bills and an overwhelming despair.

Terri's story is far from unique. Consider Mrs. Jolene Hollar of Arizona, who faced a different but equally chilling form of discrimination in 2000. Jolene applied for life insurance only to be rejected by not one but two companies. It was not because she had any illness, but because her family had a history of Huntington's disease. She hadn't even been tested for the gene herself. One insurer coldly informed her they would reconsider if she underwent testing and proved negative for the mutation. The message was clear: your genes are your destiny, whether or not you've chosen to know them.

These cases, and others like them, were precisely why the Genetic Information Nondiscrimination Act (GINA) was passed in 2008. GINA was legislation designed to address a growing fear that genetic information could become a modern-day scarlet letter. It was the first federal law to proactively protect Americans from discrimination based on their genetic makeup.

Under GINA, health insurers are prohibited from using genetic information to determine coverage or premiums, and employers are barred from considering genetic data in hiring, firing, or promotion decisions. The law encouraged people to embrace testing without the looming threat of their results being used against them.

However, while GINA was a landmark achievement, it had significant limitations. It doesn't apply to life insurance, disability insurance, or long-term care insurance. This leaves people like Jolene unprotected. Nor does it cover employers with fewer than 15 employees, creating loopholes that can leave workers vulnerable. These gaps in coverage highlight the ongoing tension between scientific progress and the ethical frameworks needed to protect individuals from harm.

Even with GINA's protections, violations persist. In 2023, Dollar General found itself in hot water for requiring job applicants to disclose detailed family medical histories during pre-employment exams. Applicants with conditions like high blood pressure or poor vision were denied job offers based on this information. The company settled with the Equal Employment Opportunity Commission, EEOC, for $1 million. This was a hefty price tag for violating GINA, but the damage to those applicants' lives had already been done.

And then there's the infamous "Devious Defecator" case; a story so absurd it borders on comedy but carries profound implications about genetic privacy. It started in 2012 at an Atlas Logistics Group warehouse in Atlanta, where someone had been leaving human feces in various locations throughout the facility. For a company specializing in grocery distribution, this was not just gross, it was catastrophically unsanitary.

Desperate to solve the mystery and restore order to their warehouse, management turned to science—or pseudoscience. They demanded cheek swabs from two employees they suspected of being the culprits. The results came back: neither man was a match. They were innocent, but by then, their dignity had been flushed away along with any trust they might have had in their employer.

Humiliated and outraged, they filed a lawsuit under GINA for the unlawful collection of their genetic data. The case went to trial in 2015 and quickly gained notoriety as *"The Devious Defecator Case."* Even the U.S. District Court Judge couldn't resist using the nickname during proceedings. It added an almost surreal layer of levity to what was otherwise a serious violation of privacy.

The jury took the matter seriously and awarded the two employees $2.25 million in damages, a landmark decision under GINA that sent shockwaves through corporate America. As for Atlas Logistics, they were left holding both a mystery and a multimillion-dollar penalty. These heartbreaking and bizarre stories are cautionary tales about what happens when genetic knowledge outpaces ethical safeguards. They remind us that while our genes may hold answers about our health and identity, they can also be used as weapons when placed in the wrong hands.

As we stand on the precipice of an era defined by genetics, the question is no longer whether genetic information will shape our future but how we will ensure it empowers rather than excludes us. Moreover, in an age of data breaches and digital surveillance, concerns about the security of information are also well-founded.

In an age of digital vulnerability, our most intimate biological information has become a tantalizing target for cybercriminals. The once-impenetrable fortress of genetic data now stands exposed, its walls breached by the relentless tide of technological advancement. With data breaches seeming so commonplace, many feel uneasy about storing their most personal biological information in databases.

This new reality has cast a shadow of unease over the promise of personalized medicine. These concerns were starkly validated in late 2023 when 23andMe, one of the world's largest genetic testing companies, suffered a massive data breach, sending waves of concern through the industry and beyond.

What began as a whisper of concern in October 2023 quickly escalated into a deafening roar of panic. The initial reports, suggesting a mere 14,000 accounts or approximately 0.1% of users, proved to be just the tip of an iceberg of unprecedented proportions. As digital forensics experts delved deeper into the breach, the devastation's true extent became horrifying: 6.9 million individuals, nearly half of 23andMe's customer base, had been exposed.

This wasn't a simple smash-and-grab hacking operation. The attackers employed a technique known as "credential stuffing," a digital battering ram that exploited an all-too-human weakness: the tendency to reuse passwords across multiple sites. Like master keys to countless genetic vaults, these stolen credentials allowed the hackers to slip past 23andMe's defenses undetected.

Once inside the system, the attackers wielded 23andMe's "DNA Relatives" feature with chilling efficiency. This tool, designed to connect users with their genetic kin, became a Pandora's box in the wrong hands. Family trees, health predispositions, and the most intimate details of gene makeup were all exposed in this digital heist.

The fallout was immediate and far-reaching. Lawsuits flooded in, forcing 23andMe to pledge $30 million to the affected individuals. But can any amount truly compensate for the loss of privacy?

The breach sent shockwaves through the industry, prompting investigations by data protection authorities in the UK and Canada. The Federal Trade Commission took unprecedented action against 1Health.io, formerly Vitagene, in 2023, marking its first case focused on the privacy and security of genetic information. The company's cavalier handling of sensitive data shocked consumers and regulators alike. Nearly 2,400 health reports and raw data of at least 227 individuals were exposed in publicly accessible "buckets" on Amazon Web Services, unencrypted and vulnerable to prying eyes.

The FTC's complaint painted a damning picture of 1Health.io's practices. Despite promising "rock-solid security," the company failed to implement essential safeguards. More egregiously, in 2020, 1Health.io retroactively expanded its data-sharing policies without notifying affected consumers or obtaining their consent, treating deeply personal genetic information as a commodity to be bartered. The $75,000 settlement and mandated security overhaul were a drop compared to the breach of trust experienced by customers who had entrusted the company with their most intimate biological data.

As the dust settled on the 1Health.io case, the genetic testing industry found itself at a crossroads, grappling with the need for a robust ethical framework to navigate the complex moral landscape of genomic medicine. The incident exposed the inadequacies of existing guidelines and highlighted the urgent need for a more comprehensive approach to ethical decision-making in this rapidly evolving field.

In response to these challenges, ethicists, researchers, and policymakers began to develop more nuanced frameworks for addressing the ethical implications of technologies. A team of experts proposed six key principles for ethical engagement in genomic research, emphasizing the importance of understanding existing regulations, fostering collaboration, building cultural competency, improving transparency, supporting capacity, and disseminating research findings. This approach aimed to build trust, increase inclusion of diverse groups, and enhance ethical research practices that respect tribal research regulations and benefit participants and their communities.

Simultaneously, genetic counselors were reevaluating their ethical guidelines, recognizing that the traditional emphasis on individual autonomy needed to be balanced with considerations of beneficence and non-maleficence. A new framework emerged, proposing six considerations for genetic counselors to weigh when deciding whether to provide recommendations to patients or families. These included the goal of counseling, clinical relevance of genetic information, informational burden of test options or results, relational considerations, role-based considerations, and familial considerations.

The genomic medicine community also grappled with the collective nature of genetic information and its implications for individual privacy and societal benefit. Some argued that patients benefiting from genome sequencing had an ethical obligation to share their health information, grounded in considerations of fairness and reciprocity. This perspective challenged traditional notions of informed consent and data ownership, suggesting that using genomic data to advance medical knowledge should be permitted without explicit consent, provided certain safeguards were in place.

As these ethical frameworks continued to evolve, they sought to balance the principles of autonomy, privacy, and confidentiality with the potential for significant societal benefits from large-scale genomic datasets. The ongoing debate underscored the need for a dynamic and adaptable ethical approach that could keep pace with rapid technological advances while upholding fundamental human rights and dignity. The tension between the promise of genetic knowledge and the fear of its misuse creates a palpable unease. We must walk carefully on this tightrope, balancing the potential for improving human health against the very real concerns about privacy and discrimination.

As genetic testing transitions from the realm of the extraordinary to the mundane, from cutting-edge science to routine medical practice, we find ourselves standing on shifting sands. The ethical and legal frameworks that once seemed adequate now creak and groan under the weight of our newfound knowledge, demanding constant reassessment and reinforcement.

Still, the promise of genetic knowledge calls us to reimagine what it means to be human, urging us to embrace a future where our genetic code is no longer a fixed destiny but a dynamic blueprint— one we can read, interpret, and... *maybe even rewrite.*

PART III

The Future of Genetic Medicine

CHAPTER 7

Beyond Disease: Enhancing Human Potential

S arah and Tom Chen sat side by side in the stark, sterile hospital waiting room, their fingers tightly interlaced, creating an unspoken bond amidst the swirling mix of excitement and anxiety that filled the air. The polished, chrome-plated walls reflected their apprehensive expressions, casting a cool, almost clinical sheen that emphasized their surroundings.

Sarah's free hand gently cradled her barely visible baby bump. This tender gesture spoke volumes about her protective instincts for the precious life blossoming within her. Every soft motion of her hand, a delicate stroke, a gentle pat, seemed to convey a silent promise of love and care as if reassuring the little one that all would be well. The weight of her expectations hung heavily in the air, mingling with the faint scent of antiseptic that permeated the room.

The soft whir of medical equipment created a rhythmic background hum, both comforting and unnerving. It summarized the blend of hope and trepidation that filled their hearts. Monitors beeped softly in synchronized intervals nearby, and the faint rustle of nurses passing in the corridor provided a fleeting distraction from their racing thoughts.

They exchanged nervous glances, each reflecting a depth of emotion: anticipation, fear, and an unshakeable commitment to each other as they embarked on this journey into parenthood. Their hearts raced with the thrill of what was to come and the weight of the uncertainties ahead. Each glance was filled with unvoiced questions and unspoken dreams. As they sat there, time seemed to stretch, yet they were united in their hope for the moment when their lives would change forever.

A holographic display flickered to life, its blue glow casting ethereal shadows across the room. It projected the image of a smiling nurse, so lifelike that for a moment, the Chens forgot it wasn't real.

"Mr. and Mrs. Chen? The doctor will see you now."

They found themselves in a pristine white room bathed in bright, sterile light as they entered the door. The air was infused with the faint scent of new plastic, creating an atmosphere that felt both clinical and avant-garde. In the center of the room stood Dr. Mohinder Suresh. He had kind, expressive eyes, a reassuring presence that instantly put them at ease. The room was filled with equipment and neatly organized workspaces. The atmosphere was charged with possibility as Dr. Suresh extended his hand in greeting, his warm smile the perfect invitation to begin their discussion.

"Congratulations on your pregnancy!" he said, his voice conveying excitement that suggested he never tired of delivering this news. "Before we begin, I have a rather important question for you both."

He held the gaze of the expectant parents, the air thick with unspoken possibilities. "Would you like to enhance or design your baby's genes?"

Tom's eyebrows shot up in surprise, a look of disbelief clouding his features. His voice wavered slightly as he asked, "Enhance? You mean like in *Gattaca*?"

Sarah's voice trembled, a flicker of uncertainty running through her as her hand instinctively tightened protectively over her barely visible baby bump. "But... isn't that playing God?" Her eyes searched Tom's, looking for reassurance amid her doubt.

Standing before them with a calm demeanor, the doctor regarded them both with understanding. "Playing God? Or perhaps it's merely playing the hand that evolution dealt us? In the past, we entrusted our children's futures to chance and uncertainty. Now, we can give them the best possible start in life."

The doctor tapped his tablet with a swift motion, and in response, a holographic DNA strand sprang to life between them. It floated effortlessly in the air, rotating slowly and casting enchanting reflections of light across the room. The vibrant colors, blues, greens, and purples, swirled and intertwined, highlighting the complex double helix structure in exquisite detail.

Each twist and turn of the strand revealed small patterns that shimmered with an ethereal quality, capturing the attention of anyone who gazed upon it. The atmosphere was one of wonder as the intricate workings of the genetic code appeared to dance gracefully before their eyes.

Tom's eyes flickered anxiously between the shimmering holographic display hovering before him and his wife's wan complexion. "But what about the risks?" he urged, his voice trembling slightly. "The ethics? The... humanity of it all?"

Dr. Suresh leaned forward, his gaze steady and piercing. The soft glow from the array of futuristic screens illuminated his salt-and-pepper hair. "The question you should be asking is:," he replied, his voice smooth yet commanding, "in a world where others are eagerly embracing these monumental advances, can you truly afford not to?" His words resonated with a relentless conviction that stirred something deep within Tom. However, doubt still lingered, thick as the tension in the room.

The future had arrived, uninvited and unannounced, thrusting them into a moral maze where the line between progress and perdition blurred with each passing heartbeat.

"So," Dr. Suresh said, his finger hovering over the tablet, ready to chart the course of human evolution, "shall we begin?"

~

While this scenario remains in the pages of sci-fi novels and on the big screen, it offers a glimpse into a rapidly approaching potential future. Are these so-called "designer babies" closer than we think?

The idea of "designer babies" has fascinated us for years. It paints a vivid picture of a future where parents can choose their child's physical attributes and cognitive traits. Imagine a world where selecting eye color, height, or intelligence becomes as commonplace as picking out a favorite outfit.

Although we haven't fully achieved this vision, recent advances in gene-editing technologies, especially CRISPR, have brought us closer to the reality of being able to change genes before a baby is born. This significant moment was notably marked in late 2018.

On November 25, a wave of astonishment rippled through the scientific community and captured the world's attention when He Jiankui, a researcher affiliated with the Southern University of Science and Technology in Shenzhen, made an unexpected announcement. He boldly proclaimed that he had successfully created the first genetically edited human babies, twin girls referred to by the pseudonyms Lulu and Nana.

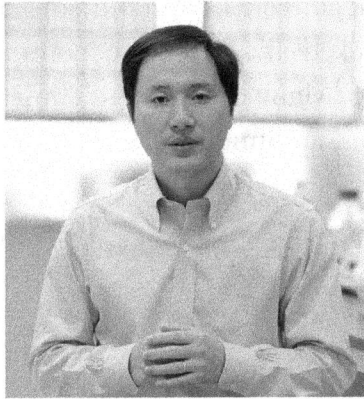

Figure 56. *He Jiankui. The He Lab*

This revelation came not through peer-reviewed scientific channels but through a series of YouTube videos bypassing scientific scrutiny and ethical oversight. He Jiankui's experiment aimed to give these children resistance to HIV by disabling the CCR5 gene, which codes for a protein that HIV uses to enter cells.

Here's how it was done: He collected sperm and eggs from couples and created embryos through *in vitro* fertilization, or IVF. Then, he used CRISPR technology to edit the embryos' genomes. Instead of replicating the natural CCR5-delta 32 mutation, He attempted to create a new mutation that would render the protein completely nonfunctional. He employed preimplantation genetic diagnosis to check for successful edits and potential errors in the embryos. The edited embryos were then implanted, resulting in the birth of twin girls.

It is important to note that while He aimed to provide resistance to HIV, his approach was flawed. The natural mutation does not confer complete protection against all forms of HIV. Furthermore, the long-term effects of this genetic modification remain unknown, raising serious ethical concerns about human germline editing. The announcement shocked the scientific community and sparked intense global debate. Many experts condemned the experiment as premature, dangerous, and unethical.

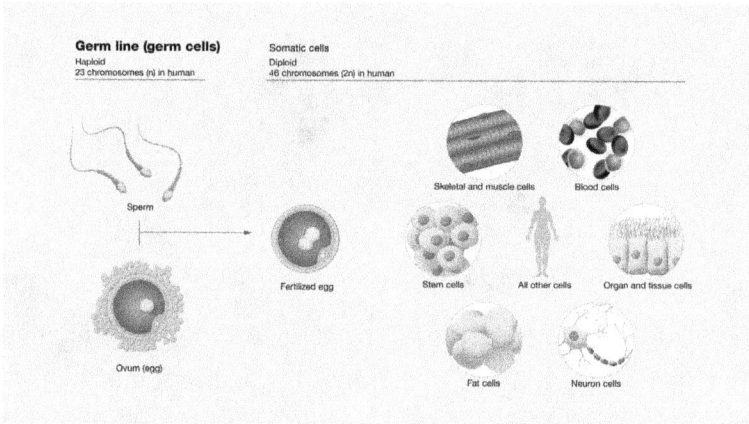

Figure 57. Germ Line. National Human Genome Research Institute

One major issue was the widespread mosaicism in both twins. Mosaicism is a condition in which an individual has two or more genetically different cell lines. In the case of the twins mentioned, not all of their cells have the same makeup. The editing process is intended to modify a specific gene related to a disease. In this case, the gene linked to HIV resistance was inconsistent throughout their bodies.

So, in simpler terms, while some cells in the twins might have the desired genetic changes, other cells might have different changes or none at all. This lack of uniformity can pose significant challenges. For instance, if the edits are meant to provide protection against disease, having a mix of edited and unedited cells can impact how effectively that protection works.

In the case of one of the twins, Lulu, He could only edit one of the two copies of the gene. This means that Lulu might have some cells with the edited version and some with the original version. As a result, she is described as "heterozygous," indicating that she has two different versions of the gene. This situation further complicates the overall effectiveness of the genetic edit, making it less predictable in terms of health outcomes.

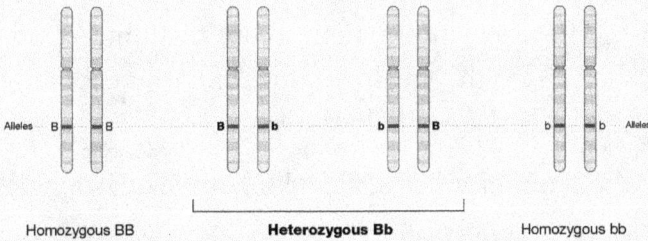

Figure 58. Heterozygous vs. homozygous. National Human Genome Research Institute

The experiment's rushed nature and lack of transparency raised serious concerns about potential off-target effects. These unintended genetic modifications could lead to significant health issues, including the risk of developing cancers or heart diseases. Moreover, there loomed the troubling prospect that these alterations might be inherited by the twins' future offspring, compounding the ethical and medical implications of the entire endeavor.

This controversial experiment thrust the debate about "designer babies" from science fiction into reality. The Chinese government placed He under police investigation and ordered his research work to be stopped. He was fired from his university position and later sentenced to three years in prison for "illegal medical practices."

The court in Shenzhen found that He and two of his collaborators had forged ethical review documents and misled doctors into unknowingly implanting gene-edited embryos into two women. During this process, it was revealed that a third genetically edited child, later identified as Amy, was born as a result of He's experiments. However, information about this third child remains limited. As of 2023, the health status and whereabouts of Lulu, Nana, and Amy are not publicly known.

The case raised numerous ethical and scientific questions. It pushed the boundaries of genetic medicine into new and uncertain areas, emphasizing the need for stricter regulations in research. It also brings forth an intricate web of ethical dilemmas that warrants careful consideration.

～୭

Picture, for a moment, a society where genetic makeup wields more influence over individual opportunities than one's geographical location or family heritage ever could. Envision yourself in a job interview, seated in a sleek, modern office, where the atmosphere is thick with expectation. As the interviewer leans forward, a seemingly casual yet provocative question slips from their lips: "Have you undergone any genetic enhancements?"

The inquiry hangs in the air, heavy with unspoken implications. A simple 'yes' or 'no' could irrevocably alter your career path, influencing decisions far beyond this initial meeting and potentially shaping your professional journey.

This unsettling scenario unfolds a chilling narrative of a new form of discrimination, wherein those who lack genetic enhancements are marginalized and relegated to the peripheries of society. These individuals are left to navigate an environment where their unmodified genetics symbolize a profound disadvantage. In this brave new world, the divide between the enhanced and the unenhanced widens.

Imagine, for a moment, a scene where hopeful parents carefully sift through a vast array of options for their unborn child, treating the selection process like a casual shopping spree. They examine choices as though they're curating a wardrobe or customizing a character in a video game, weighing every detail carefully.

Hair color? Check.

Athletic ability? Of course.

Intelligence quotient? Why not?

The pressure to create the "perfect" child becomes overwhelming, transforming the joy of parenthood into a high-stakes game of genetic roulette. Those who opt out – whether by choice or due to financial constraints – may be plagued by guilt, wondering if they've shortchanged their child's future before it even begins.

As we explore the future, we must face existential questions that were once the territory of philosophers and science fiction writers. *When does gene enhancement shift from improving the human condition to fundamentally altering what it means to be human?*

This presents a slippery slope that could lead to a future where humanity splinters into distinct subspecies, forever changing the course of our evolution. Even if we can distribute genetic enhancements fairly, a monumental challenge, we still face significant obstacles. The complex interplay between genetics and environment suggests societal inequalities could still distort the playing field.

Consider two genetically enhanced individuals: one raised in a nurturing, resource-rich environment, the other in poverty and stress. Their potential may be equal, but their life outcomes could be worlds apart. Moreover, our current gene-editing tools are far from perfect.

CRISPR-Cas9, often hailed as genetic scissors, can sometimes snip in the wrong places, potentially introducing new disorders even as it attempts to eliminate others. It's a high-stakes game of roulette, where the consequences of a misstep could echo through generations.

On a global scale, the advent of genetic technologies threatens to carve new, deeper chasms between nations. As wealthy countries race ahead, perfecting these techniques and reaping their benefits, less affluent nations risk being left behind, creating a world where one's birth determines one's opportunities and one's very potential. While the ethical debates persist, examining the real possibilities and limitations is crucial. Current research suggests that some enhancements may be more feasible than others.

～ˀ

One of the most promising frontiers in genetic enhancement is fortifying our immune systems against a wide array of pathogens.

Imagine a world where the common cold is as obsolete as smallpox and global pandemics are swiftly contained before they can wreak havoc.

At the forefront of this research is developing genetic modifications that can confer broad-spectrum viral resistance. One breakthrough, similar to the idea in the He Jiankui affair, involves a gene called C46, which has shown potential in combating HIV infection. The gene is a powerful shield against the virus when introduced into immune cells.

The C46 peptide is derived from a part of the virus's envelope glycoprotein. Essentially, it acts like a barrier that stops the HIV from entering healthy cells in our body. It does this by disrupting a crucial process that the virus needs to fuse with and invade these cells. By doing this, it can help protect our cells from an HIV infection.

Clinical trials conducted on HIV-infected patients have shown promising results regarding the safety and effectiveness of C46-modified immune cells. These positive outcomes have encouraged us to investigate further, particularly into using C46-modified stem cells. These cells give rise to all cells when treating patients with high-risk AIDS-related lymphoma.

However, enhancing the immune system is quite complex. Our immune system isn't just a straightforward line of defense; it's a sophisticated network of various cells and tissues that work together to keep us healthy. When we consider genetic modifications like the introduction of C46, they must tread carefully. While we might strengthen the immune response against one type of virus, we could inadvertently compromise our defense against another or even provoke unwanted autoimmune reactions, where the immune system might attack the body's healthy cells.

To navigate these challenges, we are pursuing multi-faceted strategies. For example, some research is exploring the combination of C46 with other anti-HIV approaches. This receptor is essential because it is one of the ways HIV enters human cells.

By using a combination of several anti-HIV methods simultaneously, the hope is to create a more formidable defense against the virus and decrease the chances of the virus developing resistance to treatment. This collaborative approach represents a hopeful pathway toward more effective therapies in the ongoing battle against HIV and possibly other viral infections.

~✲

The prospect of enhancing human intelligence through genetic modification also continues to captivate both scientists and the public imagination. While we're still far from creating "super-geniuses," we have made intriguing discoveries that hint at the potential for cognitive enhancement. One of the most promising findings involves a gene variant called KL-VS, associated with the KLOTHO gene. This variant, carried by approximately 20-25% of the population, has been linked to improved cognitive performance across various studies.

A study led by the Gladstone Institutes and the University of California, San Francisco, found that individuals carrying a single copy of the KL-VS variant performed better on a wide range of cognitive tests. Animal experiments further supported this discovery, which showed that the variant strengthened connections between neurons, enhancing synaptic plasticity—a crucial mechanism for learning and memory formation. This means that when they looked at how this works in mice, they found the variant helps strengthen the connections between brain cells. Specifically, it is crucial for learning and remembering things.

However, the relationship between KL-VS and cognitive function appears complex and potentially age-dependent. While some studies have reported cognitive benefits in younger adults and children, others have found no significant advantage or even poorer cognitive performance in older populations. For instance, a study of 1,480 Danish individuals aged 92-100 years found that KL-VS heterozygotes showed poorer cognitive function than non-carriers. This suggests that the cognitive effects of the KL-VS variant may change over the lifespan.

In simpler terms, this means that the effect of having this genetic variant can change as a person gets older. For example, while some studies have found that middle-aged adults with the variant perform better on cognitive tests, research on very old individuals, 92-100 years old, showed that those with the variant had poorer cognitive function.

Interestingly, recent research has also explored the interaction between the KL-VS variant and Alzheimer's disease pathology. A study published in 2021 found that among individuals with high levels of amyloid, a hallmark of Alzheimer's, those carrying the variant showed better cognitive performance compared to non-carriers. This suggests that the variant might offer some protection against the cognitive decline typically seen in Alzheimer's disease.

It's important to understand that a single gene does not determine intelligence and cognitive function. Instead, they result from the combined effects of many genes and environmental factors. While the KL-VS variant is an interesting piece of the puzzle, it is just one of many factors that influence cognitive abilities. We are still working to fully understand how this gene variant affects cognition and how it might be used to help people in the future.

As we unravel the genetic underpinnings of cognition, we must approach the prospect of cognitive enhancement with optimism and caution, considering the potential benefits, ethical implications, and unforeseen consequences of altering human intelligence.

The most immediately applicable and tantalizing area of genetic enhancement lies in potentially eliminating predispositions to various conditions. We have made remarkable strides in identifying genes associated with a wide range of disorders, from obesity to depression, opening up new avenues for targeted interventions.

One of the most extensively studied genes in this context is FTO, also known as the Fat Mass and Obesity-Associated gene. Variations in this have been strongly linked to an increased risk of obesity. A study from UCL, the Medical Research Council, and King's College London Institute of Psychiatry revealed why individuals with specific variants are more likely to become obese.

The research showed that people carrying the obesity-risk variant have higher circulating levels of ghrelin. Ghrelin is often referred to as the "hunger hormone." This leads to feeling hungry again soon after eating a meal. Furthermore, brain imaging revealed that the gene variation alters how the brain responds to ghrelin and food images in regions linked to eating control and reward.

Dr. Rachel Batterham, who led the study, explained in a UCL News story: "Individuals with two copies of the obesity-risk FTO variant are biologically programmed to eat more. These people have higher ghrelin levels and, therefore, feel hungrier. Still, their brains respond differently to ghrelin and to pictures of food—it's a double hit."

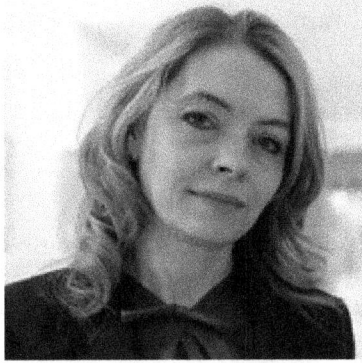

Figure 59. Rachel Batterham. University College London

This discovery provides a potential target for genetic intervention. In theory, modifying the FTO gene could reduce an individual's susceptibility to weight gain by altering their physiological response to food and hunger cues.

Similarly, genes have been linked to depression, opening up possibilities for genetic interventions in mental health. The gene is involved in the transport of serotonin. Serotonin is often called the "happy chemical" because it plays a crucial role in regulating our mood and overall sense of well-being. It's a natural substance produced by our body, primarily in the brain and gut, that acts as a messenger between nerve cells.

Serotonin acts as a tiny courier that delivers important messages throughout your body, especially in your brain. When serotonin levels are balanced, you're more likely to feel happy, calm, and focused. The gene plays a crucial role in this process by helping to control how serotonin moves around in the brain, ensuring it reaches where it's needed.

When this transport system works well, your mood tends to be more stable. This is why many antidepressants target serotonin levels or its effectiveness in the brain. However, if your body doesn't produce enough serotonin or can't use it effectively, it can lead to mood disorders like depression. Despite the importance of serotonin and the gene, it's critical to remember that most mental health conditions result from complex interactions between multiple genes and environmental factors, rather than a single genetic variation.

This underscores a critical point: modifying a single gene may not be sufficient to completely eliminate the risk of developing complex conditions. The interplay between genetics and environment is intricate and not fully understood. Recent research has also highlighted the importance of gene-environment interactions in the development of diseases.

As we unravel the complexities of genetic predispositions, it is becoming increasingly clear that the most effective strategy may be a holistic approach that combines interventions with lifestyle modifications. Eliminating genetic predispositions holds immense promise but is fraught with complexity.

We stand at a crossroads where the decisions we make today will shape the future of our species. The potential benefits are enormous: a world free from genetic diseases, enhanced resistance to viruses, and possibly even improved cognitive and physical capabilities. Yet, the risks and ethical considerations are equally significant.

As we continue to unlock the secrets of our genome, we must proceed with caution, wisdom, and a deep respect for the complexity of human biology. The future of genetic enhancement is not a distant sci-fi scenario but a rapidly approaching reality that demands our attention, understanding, and careful consideration. In fact, by 2025, precision medicine and genetic testing had already become integral parts of healthcare systems worldwide.

CHAPTER 8

From Risk to Routine: Genetic Screening

In the hushed corridors of maternity wards across America, with a single drop of blood, we stand on the precipice of unlocking the human genome's deepest secrets, rewriting the very narrative of human health. Imagine a world where a newborn's first cry is met not just with tears of joy but with a glimpse into their genetic future. A world where parents cradle not only their child but also the knowledge to shape that child's destiny.

As millions of tiny heel pricks yield their microscopic treasures, we are amassing a library of life. Each vial of newborn blood is a tome of potential, a roadmap of triumphs and challenges yet to come. In this new era, we are not merely observers of genetic fate but active participants in its unfolding story.

Public health experts recognize the long-term advantages of investing in genetic screening. Approximately 12,500 infants each year, children who might otherwise face severe disability or even death, are identified and given a chance at a healthier life. It's akin to a vaccine for the genomic age: inexpensive, universally beneficial, and incredibly effective. This progress, however, starkly contrasts with the limited options of the past.

For decades, the landscape of genetic insight was a barren one, with expectant parents navigating a treacherous path between uncertainty and invasive procedures. The tools at their disposal were crude by today's standards—either waiting for symptoms to manifest after birth or braving the risks of invasive prenatal testing.

For those seeking answers before birth, the choices were fraught with anxiety. Amniocentesis is typically performed between 15 and 20 weeks of pregnancy. During this procedure, a thin needle is inserted through the abdomen to extract a small amount of amniotic fluid containing fetal cells. It carries a risk, about 0.1-0.3%, of miscarriage.

Chorionic Villus Sampling or CVS is done earlier in pregnancy, usually between 10 and 13 weeks. It involves collecting a tiny sample of placental tissue and has a slightly higher miscarriage risk than amniocentesis, about 0.3-1%. Both procedures can diagnose chromosomal abnormalities like Down syndrome with nearly 100% accuracy, as well as many other genetic disorders.

Picture an anxious mother, her hands trembling as a needle glints under sterile lights. The amniocentesis miscarriage risk might seem small on paper, but in that cold clinic room, it looms as large as a storm cloud. These tests, while nearly flawless in accuracy, demand a Faustian bargain: risk a wanted pregnancy to safeguard it. Now, a new path emerges: non-invasive prenatal testing, or NIPT, a maternal blood test as simple as a routine checkup. No needles into the child. No risk to the child. Just answers.

This new option is a breakthrough in prenatal care. Imagine tiny fragments of fetal DNA, like whispers from the womb, circulating in the mother's bloodstream. These fragments from the placenta carry the baby's genetic makeup. With a simple blood draw from the mother, NIPT analyzes pieces of fetal DNA originating from the placenta and circulating in the mother's bloodstream. This offers a safer alternative to traditional methods, such as amniocentesis or chorionic villus sampling.

It can be performed as early as ten weeks into pregnancy when the fetus is no larger than a strawberry. At this delicate stage, when life is just beginning to take shape, this test offers an unprecedented opportunity for early intervention if needed. It also brings us one step closer to noninvasively sequencing the fetal genome.

It is exceedingly accurate in detecting common chromosomal abnormalities. This is critical because, according to the American College of Obstetricians and Gynecologists, chromosomal abnormalities affect 1 in 150 pregnancies and are also a factor in 50% of early pregnancy losses. For conditions like Down syndrome, it's like having a compass that points accurately north more than 99% of the time. It can even reveal the baby's sex with high precision.

Non-invasive prenatal testing, for all its marvels, is not a crystal ball. It cannot predict every twist and turn in a child's genetic history. Also, it's essential to understand that it's a screening test, not a definitive diagnosis. Positive results from it are like signposts pointing toward areas that need closer inspection, often leading to more traditional diagnostic tests for confirmation.

This limitation underscores an important truth: while NIPT has transformed prenatal care, it exists within a broader spectrum of genetic testing options. Its role is not to replace older methods entirely but to complement them. It offers a safer first step for families seeking answers.

Despite its relatively recent introduction, first implemented in countries like China in 2010 and publicly funded in places like the Netherlands since 2014, non-invasive prenatal testing has rapidly gained traction worldwide. In the United States, it has been routinely available since 2011. It is now recommended for all pregnant women regardless of risk factors. This widespread adoption reflects not just its scientific reliability but also its profound impact on prenatal care.

Of course, cost remains a factor in this equation. Some advanced genetic tests carry price tags of thousands of dollars, a climb not everyone can afford. Compared to standard newborn tests, non-invasive prenatal testing is generally more expensive, but this is changing. Like all genetic technologies, NIPT has seen its price decrease over time as it becomes more widespread and accessible.

Increasingly, insurance companies recognize its value in prenatal care, particularly for high-risk pregnancies. Medicaid coverage policies create a maze of accessibility. A family's zip code can determine whether they reach the summit or remain in the foothills of genetic understanding. Different states have varying Medicaid coverage policies for genetic testing and treatments, which can impact accessibility for lower-income families.

Most states charge a screening fee, typically ranging from less than $15 to nearly $60 per newborn. But here's the rub: this fee is often just a down payment on a much costlier expedition. Like a hiker realizing their map covers only the first leg of the journey, families and healthcare systems find themselves scrambling to fund the rest of the trek.

When financing a screening program, it is essential to ensure that the benefits of testing, such as early detection and treatment, outweigh the costs. Early detection can significantly improve outcomes for various health conditions by allowing timely interventions to prevent severe complications or fatalities. For example, in cases of certain congenital disorders, early screening can lead to immediate treatment options that improve the quality of life for those affected and reduce long-term healthcare costs associated with managing chronic conditions.

As the financial barriers crumble, a once-exclusive technology is becoming as accessible as a public library; a repository of genetic knowledge open to all. Like explorers standing at the edge of an uncharted map, expectant parents face a brave new world filled with promise and uncertainty.

When your child's future hangs in the balance, seeking knowledge feels less like a choice and more like an imperative, a responsibility to protect and prepare. Parents no longer must choose between ignorance and risk. Instead, they can embrace a future where genetic insights are gleaned safely, comprehensively, and as a matter of routine public health.

Every child deserves the best possible start in life, and expanded genetic screening could provide us with the tools to make that a reality. Imagine a child diagnosed with cystic fibrosis at birth who avoids years of hospitalizations thanks to early interventions. Picture a baby flagged for sickle cell anemia receiving life-altering therapies before their first birthday.

In the United States, some states offer comprehensive screening for over 100 conditions, while others provide far fewer options. This disparity creates an unsettling reality: one in which a child's access to life-saving diagnostics depends on something as arbitrary as their zip code.

Picture two newborns arriving into the world on the very same day. One baby is welcomed in North Carolina, a state with a comprehensive screening program covering over 100 medical conditions. This ensures that potential health issues are identified early on.

Meanwhile, the other baby is born in a different state with a more limited set of screenings, facing an uncertain future. While one child might be shielded from years of anguish or even a tragic fate, the other could be left to grapple with undiagnosed conditions, all dictated by the arbitrary line of geography.

This patchwork system stems from how newborn screening programs are implemented in the U.S. The Recommended Uniform Screening Panel or RUSP lists 35 core conditions and 26 secondary ones that experts agree should be screened for in every state. The RUSP is a national guideline for newborn screening established by the Advisory Committee on Heritable Disorders in Newborns and Children and approved by the Secretary of Health and Human Services.

However, these recommendations are just that—recommendations. Each state decides which conditions to include in its program, leading to significant variation in what is tested and when new conditions are added. Even when states decide to expand their screening panels, the implementation process can be painfully slow. Due to logistical hurdles or competing public health priorities, new tests can take months, or even years, to roll out. Some states may lack the financial resources to adopt new recommendations quickly. States may prioritize certain conditions based on their population's needs or the prevalence of specific disorders in their region.

This situation creates a dilemma. On one hand, state autonomy allows for tailored approaches to public health. On the other hand, it raises questions of health equity and whether a child's access to potentially life-saving screening should be determined by geographic chance.

Should a baby's chance at early detection and treatment hinge on where they happen to be born? Is it acceptable for some states to lag behind others when lives hang in the balance?

∼❧

These questions address the fundamental issue of equitable healthcare in a diverse and expansive nation. Efforts are underway to tackle these disparities. Organizations like the Association of Public Health Laboratories work to support states in expanding their screening programs. The Newborn Screening Technical Assistance and Evaluation Program, NewSTEPs, collaborates with federal agencies to improve the quality of newborn screening test results at state public health laboratories. Through its quality improvement initiatives, this program helped reduce the average time from specimen collection to result reporting by 5.2 hours.

Technological advances also hold promise. New methods are making genetic testing faster, cheaper, and more accessible than ever before. Polygenic risk scores were developed with 23% improved accuracy across diverse ancestries using multi-ethnic genomic data, but implementation remains uneven. Only 31% of Medicaid programs currently cover next-generation sequencing for newborn screening despite cost reductions from $5,000 to $100 per test over the past decade.

The 2020 revision of the Ten Essential Public Health Services framework, now with equity as its core principle, has driven programs like NorthShore's DNA-10K initiative. This model achieved 89% testing uptake across diverse populations by integrating genetic consent processes into primary care workflows. However, progress is uneven and cannot come soon enough for many families.

The challenges we face in ensuring equitable access to newborn screening in the United States are mirrored and often magnified on a global scale. Newborn screening varies significantly across countries, creating a patchwork of newborn screening practices worldwide, and the landscape is highly diverse in Europe. In July 2024, Genomics England launched the Generation Study, aiming to sequence 100,000 newborn genomes. This is a moonshot project to provide families with essential health information.

Italy performs screening for 49 conditions, while countries like the Netherlands screen for 22, Germany for 17, and Ireland for 8. France screens for only six diseases but is revisiting its strategy, while smaller countries like Liechtenstein send samples to neighboring nations for analysis. Southeastern Europe also shows disparities, with over 90% coverage in most countries but gaps in Bulgaria, Romania, and Malta.

Latin America reflects similar variability. Costa Rica leads the region by screening for 29 conditions, including congenital hypothyroidism, phenylketonuria, congenital adrenal hyperplasia, cystic fibrosis, galactosemia, hemoglobinopathies, and metabolic disorders. Mexico screens for 6 to 76 disorders, depending on the healthcare system, while Argentina, Brazil, and Cuba screen for six conditions. Some countries, like El Salvador, only screen for congenital hypothyroidism, leaving millions of newborns without access to comprehensive screening programs.

In Asia and the Middle East, progress is uneven. China screens over 90% of its approximately 12 million annual births using a national panel that regions can expand. Singapore has incorporated SCID into its national panel in Southeast Asia. At the same time, other countries are lagging.

The Middle East has shown promise, with Qatar screening all newborns for spinal muscular atrophy since 2021. Lebanon has pioneered SCID screening in the region. Africa faces significant challenges in newborn screening coverage. With approximately 30 million births annually, fewer than 1 million babies are screened yearly due to limited infrastructure and resources.

Globally, only about 28% of the 140 million babies born annually receive some form of newborn screening. This disparity underscores differences in healthcare systems, economic resources, and regional public health priorities. As technology advances and awareness grows, there is hope for more comprehensive and standardized practices worldwide. This offers millions of children a healthier start to life and reshapes global healthcare outcomes for future generations. These global statistics aren't just numbers; they represent real children and families who are either given a chance at a healthier life or are left to face potentially preventable health challenges.

As our understanding of the human genome deepens, the complexity of genetic tests has skyrocketed, leading to new challenges. Misinterpretation of results can lead to unnecessary anxiety, overtreatment, or even misdiagnosis. For example, there have been cases where a variant of uncertain significance was initially interpreted as high-risk, causing months of worry before further analysis revealed it to be benign. Variants of uncertain significance are genetic changes detected during newborn screening that lack sufficient evidence to determine whether they are harmful or benign. These ambiguous results are surprisingly common.

In X-linked adrenoleukodystrophy, screening programs have shown that 62% of missense variants initially classified as pathogenic were later reclassified as variants of uncertain significance due to a lack of understanding of their clinical implications. Similarly, in Michigan's biotinidase deficiency program, 84.5% of screen-positive cases involved partial enzyme deficiencies with unclear prognoses, leaving families in a state of diagnostic uncertainty.

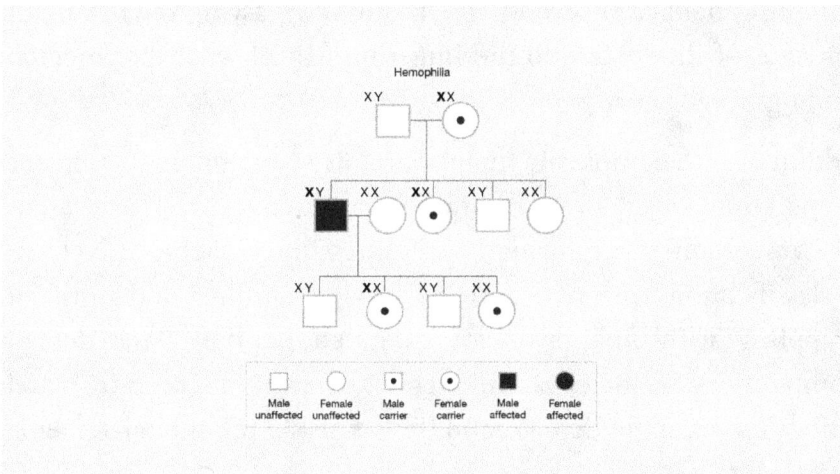

Figure 60. X-linked disease. National Human Genome Research Institute

For cystic fibrosis, inconclusive results labeled as "cystic fibrosis screen positive, but inconclusive diagnosis" have now outnumbered classic cystic fibrosis diagnoses in certain regions. The ratios vary significantly, ranging from 1.2:1 in Poland to 32:1 in Ireland. This indicates a growing trend in inconclusive test results that may reflect differences in screening practices or genetic factors within these populations.

The uncertainty surrounding these results can have profound effects on families. Parents often face months, or even years, of waiting for follow-up tests and reanalysis, which can prolong anxiety and confusion. In some cases, invasive confirmatory testing, such as skin biopsies for enzyme assays, is required to resolve uncertainty.

The psychological toll is significant; mothers of infants with inconclusive results report higher levels of perceived uncertainty compared to those whose children receive definitive diagnoses. Interviews with families reveal that parents develop hypervigilant parenting behaviors, excessively monitoring asymptomatic infants for signs of illness due to the lingering fear of what the uncertain findings might mean.

Adding to the complexity, many variants of uncertain significance remain unresolved for years. Studies show that only 7.3% of variants of uncertain significance interpretations achieve clinical reclassification within two years, leaving families and clinicians grappling with unknowns for extended periods. This delay is compounded by the expanding scope of newborn screening panels, which increasingly detect conditions outside traditional screening parameters.

Genomic sequencing can identify genetic changes, but many alterations do not have clinical significance. Although advances in technology have made genetic testing quicker and more affordable, reducing costs from $1 million in 2007 to just $600 today, these innovations also create new challenges in interpreting complex findings.

Using the complex results of newborn screening is a delicate balance. On one hand, early detection can save lives by enabling timely treatment for severe conditions. On the other hand, presenting uncertain findings without clear guidance risks causing unnecessary anxiety and harm to families. We want to provide as much information as possible. Still, we also need to be careful about presenting uncertain findings.

It's critical to remember these are not just statistics—they are real families.

Consider Nora Eysen, diagnosed with Infantile Onset Pompe Disease just two weeks after birth. Without early detection, this rare and life-threatening condition could have claimed her life. Instead, prompt medical intervention has transformed her prognosis, allowing her to blossom into a lively three-year-old. Her mother eloquently captures the profound impact of newborn screening: *"It gave us our best possible outcome."*

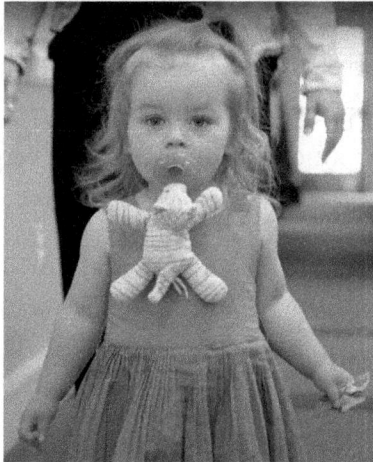

Figure 61. *Nora Eysen. Greenwood Genetic Center*

For the Mays family, newborn screening was lifesaving. Their daughter Indie was diagnosed with Maple Syrup Urine Disease, a rare metabolic disorder that, if undetected, can cause irreversible brain damage. Thanks to early intervention and a carefully managed diet, Indie now has the chance to lead a healthy and fulfilling life—a future that might have been lost without this critical test.

Not every journey is straightforward, however. Henry Whyte's story underscores the disparities in global healthcare access. His family faced significant challenges securing specialized care while living in Dubai, highlighting the urgent need for equitable newborn screening programs and follow-up care worldwide.

These narratives paint a vivid picture of newborn screening's impact: lives saved, families spared from heartache, and children given the chance to thrive against incredible odds. Each heel prick represents not just a test, but a gateway to possibility. This is a chance to rewrite genetic destinies and offer hope where once there might have been only uncertainty.

Many people who could benefit from this knowledge remain excluded from its advantages. Genetic screening stands out as a beacon of potential, promising a future where every child's health story begins with understanding. However, this promising opportunity is entangled in a web of challenges.

This raises an important question: *why, in an age of remarkable medical advances, do we still struggle to make this life-changing technology accessible to everyone who needs it?*

~❧

Several factors contribute to this underuse. One major issue is the significant lack of awareness among the public and healthcare providers. There is a pervasive fog within the public and medical communities alike.

Many healthcare providers stand at the edge of this frontier, unequipped to navigate the labyrinth of genetic risk. A study of electronic health records found that among 299 randomly selected women receiving care in the UW Medicine system, only 24 were identified as meeting guidelines for risk assessment. This suggests a substantial gap in recognizing candidates for genetic testing.

Physicians also hesitate to order tests they can't interpret, leaving patients adrift in a sea of unanswered questions. The reluctance is not unfounded; studies reveal significant gaps in confidence among nongenetic professionals regarding testing. 43% of medical professionals lack confidence in interpreting genetic test results. Additionally, 56% are uncertain about the types of tests available. Even more concerning, 62% struggle to identify which are appropriate for their patients. Furthermore, 45% feel unprepared to make treatment recommendations based on test results.

Additionally, many providers are not confident or feel unprepared to work with patients at high risk for genetic conditions, making it difficult for them to interpret test results effectively. Primary care physicians reported low confidence in ordering testing for hereditary cancers, with only 23.8% feeling confident in this task.

For families, the problem is more straightforward yet more devastating: they simply don't know these tests *exist*. A study published in the *Journal of Community Genetics* found that only 56% of participants had heard of genetic testing for cancer risk. Also, many don't understand how they could affect their health. Imagine a parent cradling a child with a rare disorder, unaware that a simple screening could have rewritten their story years earlier.

Access is another barrier to expanded screening. As of 2017, 49% of genetic counselors in the United States were concentrated in just ten states: California, New York, Pennsylvania, Texas, Massachusetts, Ohio, Illinois, Michigan, North Carolina, and Minnesota.

This concentration creates a landscape where genetic counselors and specialized clinics become modern-day oases in a vast healthcare desert. In cities, these services thrive as bustling hubs where hope and science converge. A study of genetic counselor distribution in the United States found that 66% of respondents worked in large cities such as New York City, Boston, and Chicago.

However, the picture changes dramatically as one ventures beyond urban areas. The landscape turns barren, with rural regions facing severe shortages in genetic services. Children from rural areas are less likely to receive recommended genetic services, and there is a roughly 600% disparity in access to child health physicians across the United States.

Access remains a challenge even in well-served urban areas due to overwhelming demand. Long waiting lists for genetic services often stretch like mirages, always visible but seemingly out of reach. In urban centers, patients usually wait 6 to 12 months for their first appointment with a genetic specialist. The journey doesn't end there; after the initial consultation, families may wait an additional 2 to 3 months for genetic test results and a final diagnosis.

Beyond geographical and capacity issues, other factors further complicate access to genetic services. Insurance coverage plays a crucial role as well. Compared to those with insurance, uninsured children were 55% less likely to access services. Income disparities also affect access, with children from high-income families being twice as likely to access genetic services.

Innovative approaches are being explored in response to these challenges. A pilot study by Children's Mercy Research Institute in Kansas City, Missouri, implemented a direct-to-provider model in partnership with a rural clinic. This approach more than doubled the historical rate of rare disease diagnosis among the rural population. It cut the time to diagnosis by about five months.

Despite such encouraging initiatives, the overall picture remains one of stark contrasts. The combination of geographical isolation, workforce shortages, and systemic barriers continues to create a significant divide in access to genetic healthcare across the United States. Addressing these disparities will require concerted efforts to expand services, increase workforce distribution, and implement innovative care delivery models.

Scaling these efforts requires more than ambition; it demands transformation. Healthcare systems must evolve to meet the increased demand for genetic insights. Providers need training to interpret complex results and communicate them effectively and compassionately to families who may feel overwhelmed by this new frontier of information. Support services, such as genetic counseling, will be vital guides for parents navigating the intricate terrain of their child's genetic map.

And what of the adults among us whose genetic secrets remain locked away in the vaults of their DNA?

~✤

While prenatal and newborn screening have transformed early detection and intervention, adult genetic testing is carving its own path through the landscape of modern medicine. Like explorers venturing into uncharted territory, individuals can now uncover hidden truths about their health risks, ancestry, and lifestyle factors. Direct-to-consumer, or DTC, genetic testing companies have opened doors to this library, allowing anyone with a simple cheek swab or vial of saliva to gain insights into their genetic predispositions.

However, it's crucial to approach DTC genetic testing with a discerning eye. As discussed earlier, privacy and security concerns loom like storm clouds on the horizon. Moreover, the results of these tests often lack the depth and clinical validation necessary for medical decision-making. They can provide a starting point, a genetic compass, but are rarely sufficient to chart a complete course through one's health journey.

Clinical genetic testing offers a robust alternative for those seeking more reliable and actionable insights. Unlike direct-to-consumer tests, these are conducted under the guidance of healthcare professionals and often include consultations with genetic counselors. Clinical tests are tailored to specific medical concerns, whether diagnosing a suspected condition, assessing cancer risk, or evaluating hereditary factors for cardiovascular disease.

Diagnostic testing becomes crucial for individuals exhibiting symptoms that whisper of a genetic disorder. This focused approach allows healthcare providers to achieve accurate diagnoses, guide treatment options, and illuminate potential risks for patients and their families. It's like spotlighting a specific chapter in one's genetic story.

Carrier screening, particularly valuable for those planning to start a family, is akin to peering into the future. It helps determine whether individuals carry genes associated with inherited conditions such as cystic fibrosis or Tay-Sachs disease. This knowledge empowers prospective parents to make informed decisions about their family's health.

Next-generation sequencing, sometimes called NGS, has emerged as the cornerstone of modern genetic medicine. It enables us to decode biological systems with unprecedented resolution. This transformative technology operates like a literary speedreader, devouring millions of DNA fragments. It's as if we've graduated from painstakingly copying texts by hand to printing entire libraries in the blink of an eye.

This style of sequencing is often called high-throughput sequencing. It dramatically increases the volume of data generated compared to newborn screening. Introduced commercially around 2005, NGS employs a massively parallel sequencing technique that allows the analysis of entire genomes or large panels of genes in a single breathtaking run. It can sequence hundreds to thousands of fragments simultaneously, starkly contrasting traditional methods that plodded along one fragment at a time.

NGS leverages sequencing-by-synthesis chemistry, where fluorescently tagged nucleotides are incorporated into growing DNA strands and imaged in real-time. This approach contrasts starkly with Sanger sequencing, which struggled with throughput limitations and exorbitant costs. A single NGS run can now generate terabytes of data, sequencing entire human genomes in days; a task that once took years and cost $3 billion during the Human Genome Project.

The cost of genome sequencing has plummeted dramatically as a stone dropped from a great height. In 2007, sequencing a human genome cost approximately $1 million; by 2025, this figure has plunged to as low as $600 per genome, thanks to advances in chemistry, imaging, and fierce competition among technology providers.

Next-gen sequencing involves several key steps: DNA samples are fragmented into smaller pieces and tagged with adapters during library preparation. These fragments are then amplified to ensure sufficient material for sequencing before being processed through advanced fluidic systems that add nucleotides one by one to growing DNA strands. Sophisticated imaging techniques capture this process in real-time, generating massive datasets that reconstruct the original genetic sequence.

This sequencing offers two main approaches: whole-genome sequencing and whole-exome sequencing. Whole-genome sequencing is like reading an entire book, while whole-exome sequencing focuses on just the most important chapters.

It sequencing examines all 3 billion letters in our DNA "book," including both the parts that directly code for proteins, exons, and the parts in between, introns. This comprehensive approach has several advantages. It provides more even coverage of our genetic information, like having consistent lighting while reading every page. Studies show that whole genome sequencing has a more balanced distribution of how deeply it reads each part of the DNA, with most areas being read about 38 times for accuracy.

Whole-genome sequencing is also better at detecting genetic variations. It misses fewer significant changes, catching about 3% more potentially harmful variations in coding regions that whole-exome sequencing might overlook. It's like having a more thorough proofreader who catches subtle typos others might miss. Whole genome sequencing is also superior at detecting large-scale changes in DNA, such as when chunks are duplicated or deleted.

On the other hand, whole-exome sequencing zeroes in on just the exons – the parts of our DNA that directly code for proteins. These comprise only 1-2% of our genome but contain most changes known to cause diseases. Whole-exome sequencing is like focusing on the most crucial chapters of our DNA book. It's generally cheaper than whole-genome sequencing. It simplifies the analysis process, making it easier for us to interpret the results.

Whole-genome sequencing performed best when compared to standard tests in children with suspected genetic disorders. It diagnoses about 41% of cases, compared to 36% for whole-exome sequencing and only 11% for standard tests. Whole-genome sequencing also slightly edged out the others in terms of clinical usefulness, helping guide medical decisions in about 74% of cases, compared to 72% for whole-exome sequencing and 69% for standard tests.

A detailed study comparing whole-exome sequencing and whole-genome sequencing in six individuals found that whole-genome sequencing identified an average of 692 high-quality genetic variations that whole-exome sequencing missed. In contrast, whole-exome sequencing only found 105, which the entire genome sequencing missed. Whole-exome sequencing also had a higher rate of false positives, 78% compared to 17% for whole-genome sequencing. This means that whole-exome sequencing is more likely to flag a change that isn't there incorrectly.

These next-generation tests have transformed medicine, enabling comprehensive genomic analyses that inform diagnoses, prognoses, and therapeutic strategies. It's like having a high-powered microscope that can zoom in on the tiniest details of our genetic makeup.

Institutions like the Mayo Clinic and Johns Hopkins Institute of Genetic Medicine use it to diagnose rare genetic conditions, analyzing complete DNA sets rather than isolated regions. This technology identifies tumor mutations, tracks cancer evolution through liquid biopsies, and guides immunotherapy decisions based on tumor mutational burden.

Interestingly, this is not all we can use this screening information for; we can also use it for what is known as pharmacogenomics.

~✿

Pharmacogenomics enables us to predict how an individual will respond to a specific medication based on their genetic profile. This precision means that the traditional "one size fits all" approach is becoming outdated. Instead, we can customize medical therapies to match each person's unique characteristics.

Take the CYP2C19 gene, for example. This is essential in creating an enzyme that helps our bodies break down a wide array of drugs. This includes several commonly prescribed antidepressants. Differences in the gene can significantly impact how someone processes these drugs.

Imagine two people who look exactly alike on the outside, both receiving the same antidepressant medication at the exact dosage. Despite their identical appearances and prescriptions, their bodies function very differently. Each person has a unique 'chemical laboratory' that processes the medication differently, leading to varying effects and outcomes.

One possesses a "rapid metabolizer" version of CYP2C19, their cellular machinery working overtime, breaking down the medication ruthlessly. For this person, the standard dose of antidepressant is like a raindrop in the ocean, broken down and swept away before it can exert its therapeutic effect. The result? A treatment rendered ineffective, leaving the patient struggling with symptoms they hoped to alleviate.

Now, consider the other individual carrying a "poor metabolizer" variant of CYP2C19. In their biochemical cityscape, the drug-processing machinery moves at a glacial pace. The antidepressant, instead of being efficiently metabolized, begins to accumulate. Slowly, at first, then with increasing speed, the medication builds up to potentially toxic levels. What was meant to be a healing balm becomes a potential poison, its concentration rising dangerously high, threatening to unleash a cascade of severe side effects.

Two patients: the exact diagnosis and prescription, yet wildly different outcomes. One left without relief, the other at risk of harm—all because of a subtle variation in a single gene.

This is where the power of pharmacogenomics truly shines. By understanding a patient's CYP2C19 status, we can look into the future to predict how a medication might perform in an individual's unique biochemical environment. With this understanding, we can customize prescriptions, much like a master chef adjusts a recipe to suit a diner's taste.

However, the implications of this genetic insight extend far beyond antidepressants. Consider the HLA-B*1502 gene, a key player in the complex orchestra of our immune system. For most people, it hums along quietly in the background. But for some, particularly those of Asian descent, it holds a potentially deadly secret.

In this context, the story of Mei, a young woman seeking relief from epilepsy, serves as a poignant example. In the sterile examination room, Mei sits, her hands trembling beneath the harsh fluorescent lights. At 23, she should be in the prime of her youth, but epilepsy has cast a dark shadow over her dreams. Each seizure comes without warning, a terrifying reminder of her fragility, leaving her exhausted and afraid.

Her doctor considers prescribing carbamazepine, a common anticonvulsant. As he explains the potential benefits, Mei allows herself to imagine a life free from the constant fear of seizures. She envisions walking confidently down the street, no longer afraid of collapsing at any moment, helpless and vulnerable.

But as Mei reached for the prescription, an unseen specter loomed over her. Unbeknownst to both doctor and patient, Mei carried a genetic variant that turned this promise of healing into a potential death sentence. Hidden within the intricate coils of Mei's DNA, the variant lay in wait, a silent time bomb. This difference, more common in individuals of Asian descent, held the power to transform carbamazepine from a healing balm into a devastating toxin.

The clock began ticking as Mei left the clinic, prescription in hand. Days passed, and Mei started her treatment, hoping to blossom in her chest. But deep within her body, an insidious process had begun. Her immune system, triggered by the interaction between carbamazepine and her HLA-B*1502 variant, was preparing for war against an enemy that didn't exist.

The first signs were subtle - a slight rash, easily dismissed as a common side effect. But within hours, Mei's world exploded into agony. Once smooth and unblemished, her skin began to blister and peel away in sheets as if she were being flayed alive. The pain was excruciating, every movement a torment as her body turned against itself in a catastrophic overreaction known as Stevens-Johnson syndrome.

As Mei fought for her life, her family huddled in the waiting room, their faces etched with horror and grief. *How could a medication meant to heal have caused such devastation?*

The answer lay hidden in her genes, a cruel twist of fate that could have been avoided with a simple test. In that heart-wrenching moment, the truth hit like a thunderclap: what if a test had illuminated the variations that made Mei vulnerable to the very treatment designed to save her?

In an alternate reality, the physician pauses instead of reaching for the prescription pad. Instead, they order a genetic test. A simple cheek swab to unlock critical insights into Mei's makeup. The test revealed Mei's HLA-B*1502 status, which was crucial information that changed everything. Armed with this knowledge, they avoided carbamazepine, choosing instead a safer alternative that wouldn't trigger Mei's genetic predisposition to a catastrophic reaction.

In this version of events, Mei leaves the clinic with a different prescription and a future full of hope. She'll never know how close she came to a life-altering tragedy, all thanks to the power of genetic insight and personalized medicine.

The implications of pharmacogenomics ripple outward, touching every corner of medicine. Imagine a future where a patient's profile is as fundamental to prescribing as their age or weight, where the trial-and-error approach to finding the proper medication gives way to precision targeting guided by each individual's unique map.

In oncology, genetic testing could predict which chemotherapy drugs will be most effective and least toxic for each cancer patient.

It could guide the choice and dosage of blood thinners for heart disease, potentially preventing life-threatening complications. In pain management, it could help navigate the treacherous waters of opioid prescribing, identifying patients at higher risk for addiction or adverse reactions.

This is the promise of pharmacogenomics: a future where medications are finely tuned tools calibrated to each person's makeup. It's a vision of healthcare where the right drug at the correct dose is not a matter of chance but a carefully calculated decision based on the most fundamental blueprint of our bodies—our DNA.

Advances in artificial intelligence and machine learning are also on the verge of transforming data interpretation by helping to prioritize clinically actionable variants from the millions produced in each genome. These technologies enhance data interpretation, improve variant prioritization, and accelerate the integration of genomic information into clinical practice.

AI algorithms are significantly enhancing the accuracy of next-generation sequencing technologies. At the forefront is NVIDIA, a company known for its graphics processing units, now powering both short- and long-read sequencing platforms with AI-accelerated base calling and variant analysis. This leap in technology is not just about speed; it's about reliability. Improving base calling accuracy leads to more dependable genomic data, a critical factor for clinical applications where lives hang in the balance.

But the true marvel lies in the scale at which AI operates. These intelligent systems can now process vast amounts of sequencing data, identifying genetic variants with a precision once thought impossible. Picture a scientist sifting through millions of genetic markers, looking for the proverbial needle in a haystack. Now, imagine that same task being completed in a fraction of the time, with even greater accuracy. This is the power of AI in genomics, dramatically reducing the time and resources required for large-scale genomic studies.

Companies like Oxford Nanopore Technologies are further changing genomic analysis. They have pushed the boundaries of read length, enabling real-time, portable sequencing. When coupled with AI algorithms, this advance allows for on-the-fly analysis of genomic data.

Envision a critically ill patient arriving at the emergency room. In the past, genetic testing could take days or weeks. This is precious time the patient might not have. Now, with AI-assisted real-time sequencing, doctors can potentially obtain crucial genetic information within hours, enabling rapid diagnosis and tailored treatment plans. This capability is particularly valuable in time-sensitive clinical scenarios, where every moment counts.

One of AI's most profound contributions to genomics is its ability to prioritize clinically actionable variants from the millions produced in each genome. Tools like Google's DeepVariant employ deep learning to identify genetic variants with greater accuracy than traditional methods. This is not just an incremental improvement; it's a quantum leap in our ability to interpret the human genome.

Moreover, AI models can now analyze polygenic risk scores to predict an individual's susceptibility to complex diseases, such as diabetes and Alzheimer's. This advance allows for more precise risk assessment and early intervention strategies, potentially saving countless lives through preventive care.

AI algorithms shine particularly bright in the realm of rare diseases. They excel at identifying rare variants that conventional analysis methods might overlook. This capability is crucial for diagnosing rare genetic disorders, especially in neonatal care, where rapid whole-genome sequencing can be the difference between life and death.

AI is not just improving our understanding of genomics in isolation; it's facilitating the integration of genomics with other 'omics' data, including transcriptomics, proteomics, metabolomics, and epigenomics. This multi-omics approach provides a more comprehensive view of biological systems, linking genetic information with molecular function and phenotypic outcomes.

Imagine peering into the intricate dance of molecules within a cell, understanding not just the genetic blueprint but how it interacts with the environment to produce the symphony of life. By analyzing this complex data, AI helps us unravel complex disease mechanisms. In cancer research, for instance, multi-omics approaches aided by AI can dissect the tumor microenvironment, revealing the intricate interactions between cancer cells and their surroundings.

The impact of AI extends beyond diagnosis and into treatment. AI analysis of genomic data accelerates the identification of new drug targets, streamlining the drug development pipeline. This approach can lead to more effective and targeted therapies, potentially changing treatment for various diseases.

In pharmacogenomics, AI-driven analyses predict how variations influence drug metabolism, allowing for optimized dosage and minimized side effects. This personalization of drug treatments is not just a scientific achievement; it's a cornerstone of medicine that promises to tailor treatments to each individual's unique genetic makeup.

The impact of AI is particularly profound in oncology. AI-assisted genomic analysis helps identify somatic mutations, structural variations, and gene fusions in tumors, paving the way for truly personalized cancer treatments. Imagine a future where each cancer patient receives a treatment plan as unique as their own DNA, targeting the specific mutations driving their disease.

As AI models become more complex, ensuring their interpretability becomes crucial, especially in clinical settings where understanding the rationale behind predictions can be a matter of life and death. We must strive for AI systems that not only provide accurate results. Still, we can also explain their reasoning in ways medical professionals can understand and trust.

While genome sequencing costs have decreased dramatically, further reductions are expected. AI-powered tools contribute to this trend by improving data processing and analysis efficiency. As costs continue to fall, the dream of routine whole-genome sequencing as part of standard medical care comes closer to reality.

The marriage of AI and genomics is not just advancing our understanding of the human genome; it's changing healthcare, drug discovery, and our very conception of what it means to be human. As we continue to unlock the secrets hidden in our DNA, we stand on the threshold of a new era. An era where treatments are tailored to our makeup, where diseases can be predicted and prevented before they manifest, and where the code of life becomes an open book, ready to be read and understood like never before.

Each ripple in this genomic sea tells a story—a tale of migration, adaptation, and survival etched into the very fabric of our being. The human genome, once a mysterious cipher, now unfolds before us like an ancient map, its contours revealing the shared odyssey of our species and the unique journeys of populations across the globe.

~⁓

Imagine, if you will, a quilt woven from the threads of six billion lives. Each strand, a genetic signature, intertwines with others, thus creating patterns of breathtaking complexity. From the neon-lit streets of Tokyo to the lush, emerald depths of the Amazon rainforest, these patterns shift and evolve, reflecting the myriad environments that have shaped human evolution. Like a kaleidoscope turning in the light, our genetic diversity dazzles with its endless variations while hinting at the shared origins that unite us all.

Yet beneath this diversity lies a profound unity—a reminder that we are all, in the end, cut from the same genetic cloth. This unity is encoded in the double helix of DNA. This universal language binds humanity together even as it celebrates our differences. It is a language written in just four letters yet capable of composing infinite stories. These stories are etched into every cell of our bodies, whispering tales of resilience, migration, adaptation, and survival.

But this genetic mosaic is far more than an abstract wonder; it is a treasure trove of insights waiting to be unlocked. Hidden within are answers to some of medicine's most perplexing mysteries.

Why, for instance, does type 2 diabetes disproportionately affect South Asian communities? Why do specific populations respond differently to medications or exhibit varying susceptibility to diseases like asthma or cancer?

These questions find their roots in our DNA: a legacy of ancient adaptations now grappling with modern lifestyles. At its core, genetic diversity refers to the variation in DNA sequences among individuals within a population. This variation shapes everything from physical traits like height and skin color to disease susceptibility and treatment response.

For instance, diversity within the Major Histocompatibility Complex, a region critical for immune system functioning, has been linked to enhanced disease resistance in both humans and animals. Nature has equipped us with an arsenal of genetic tools, each uniquely suited to help us survive in different environments.

However, this diversity is not guaranteed. Like a forest that thrives on biodiversity but falters when reduced to monoculture, human populations with low genetic variation face significant health risks. Research has shown that reduced diversity, often caused by population bottlenecks or inbreeding, can increase susceptibility to conditions like high blood pressure, asthma, and infectious diseases such as tuberculosis and hepatitis. This highlights why preserving genetic diversity is not just important, it's essential for our collective health and survival.

The advent of personalized or precision medicine has transformed how we think about healthcare. Precision medicine aspires to replace the "one-size-fits-all" approach with therapies as personalized as fingerprints by tailoring treatments to an individual's unique makeup. However, this ambitious vision hinges on understanding the full spectrum of human diversity.

Take Africa, the cradle of humanity, as an example. The continent boasts unparalleled genetic diversity, with variations more than 200 times greater than those observed in other world populations. This diversity offers immense opportunities for advancing precision medicine but also presents challenges when standardizing drug use across varied genetic landscapes.

A recent study examining populations in southern and southwestern China has provided valuable insights into genetic diversity and carrier status in these regions. Expanded carrier screening analyzed 220 diseases among 3,024 individuals. They found a carrier frequency for pathogenic or likely pathogenic variants of 62.3%. Notably, 23.2% of the individuals were identified as carriers of multiple diseases, with each subject carrying an average of 0.938 pathogenic or likely pathogenic variants.

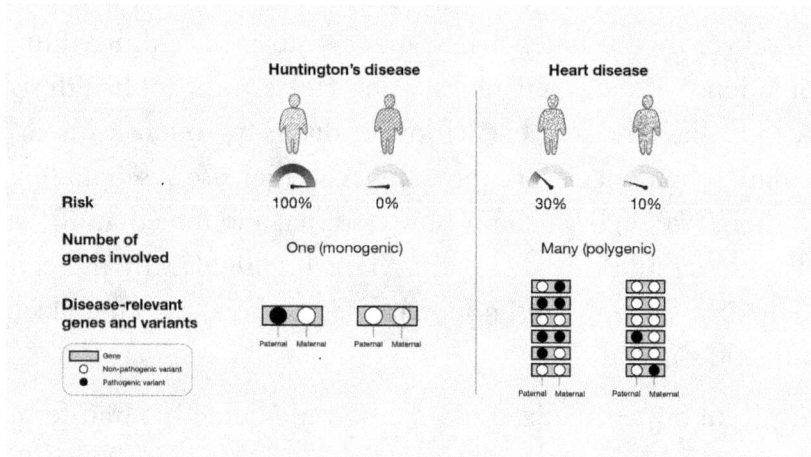

Figure 62. Example of Pathogenic Variants. National Human Genome Research Institute

Additionally, the study identified 128 at-risk couples who carried pathogenic or likely pathogenic variants of the same gene. This suggests a theoretical incidence rate of 2.12% for these variants in their offspring. These findings highlight the importance of comprehensive genetic screening in diverse populations, as it can provide crucial information for reproductive guidance and the early detection of genetic disorders.

These efforts face significant challenges: harmonizing data collection methods across countries is no small feat, especially when navigating varying ethical and regulatory frameworks. Ensuring equitable benefit-sharing from research findings requires trust-building through community engagement and moral transparency. Moreover, underrepresentation and ancestral bias in research continue to skew our understanding of disease genetics.

Many genomic studies have predominantly used data from individuals of European descent. This reliance has resulted in predictive models that often do not work well for underrepresented populations, and such bias distorts research findings. It perpetuates health disparities by providing less effective treatments to non-European groups.

As of 2016, over 80% of participants in genome-wide association studies were of European descent, even though this group represents only about 7% of the global population. This imbalance leads to health disparities by limiting the applicability of findings for non-European populations. For instance, risk models created from predominantly European data often perform poorly when applied to other groups, resulting in inaccurate diagnoses and ineffective treatments. Indigenous peoples and individuals from low- and middle-income countries are especially at risk of exclusion due to logistical challenges or historical mistrust of biomedical research.

Large-scale international initiatives, such as the 1000 Genomes Project and H3Africa, are stepping up to address these challenges by mapping genetic variation across diverse populations. The 1000 Genomes Project, one of the most ambitious efforts in genomics, seeks to catalog variations from populations worldwide. This initiative provides us with a comprehensive reference of human genetic diversity, enabling us to identify variants associated with diseases and traits across different ancestries.

Similarly, H3Africa focused on studying the genomes of African populations, which harbor the greatest genetic diversity on Earth. This diversity reflects the continent's role as the cradle of humanity. It offered insights into disease mechanisms and evolutionary biology.

These initiatives empower individuals by providing knowledge about their genetic predispositions, such as an increased risk for heart disease or unique responses to specific medications. With this information, healthcare providers can develop personalized intervention strategies that emphasize proactive care, preventing diseases before they occur, rather than reactive medicine, which focuses on treating illnesses after they have arisen.

As we delve deeper into the genetic landscape, we find ourselves on the cusp of a new era where personalized medicine reigns supreme. This approach transcends traditional "one-size-fits-all" methods, allowing for treatments that are intricately tailored to each individual's unique makeup. Picture a healthcare system where your medical care is as distinctive as your fingerprint, with every treatment plan crafted with the precision of a bespoke suit, fitted perfectly to your specific needs and characteristics.

As we embrace this new era of genetic awareness and testing, the question arises: *What practical steps do we need to take? How do we gather and harness this medical information on a large scale and then apply it to save and transform lives worldwide?*

CHAPTER 9

The Future Is in Our Genes

The genetic revolution is no longer a distant promise—*it's here*, reshaping medicine and redefining what's possible for human health. For patients tethered to chronic treatments, gene therapy offers something almost unimaginable: *freedom*.

It can cure untreatable diseases and replace a lifetime of invasive care with a single transformative treatment. But this promise comes with a staggering price tag, raising urgent questions about who will benefit *and who might be left behind*.

Consider Hemgenix, priced at $3.5 million per treatment for hemophilia B. In this genetic bleeding disorder, patients lack a crucial blood clotting protein. Zolgensma, previously the most expensive drug at $2.1 million per dose, treats spinal muscular atrophy, a rare condition affecting muscle strength. Zynteglo, priced at $2.8 million, offers a one-time treatment for beta-thalassemia patients, potentially freeing them from lifelong blood transfusions. The lifetime cost of Vyjuvek, a topical gene therapy for dystrophic epidermolysis bullosa, could be up to $15-$22 million per patient.

The considerable expense associated with cell and gene therapies is apparent. According to a report in *Nature* that analyzed gene therapies approved by December 2020 and those in advanced clinical trials, the average annual cost of these therapies is around

$20.4 billion. The report forecasts that this expenditure will increase to $25.3 billion by 2026 before tapering off to $21.0 billion by 2034.

These high costs create an uncomfortable paradox. While these therapies promise to reduce long-term healthcare costs by eliminating chronic treatments, their upfront prices make them inaccessible for many patients and unsustainable for healthcare systems already under strain.

The urgency of these challenges cannot be overstated. Gene therapy represents one of the most transformative advances in modern medicine. A *chance to rewrite the futures of millions of people living with rare or debilitating conditions.* Its success depends on scientific breakthroughs, bold thinking, and collective action across governments, industries, and communities. This chapter isn't just about numbers or policy debates—it's about the future we want to build.

Imagine a child born in a rural town with a rare genetic disorder. Her parents learn that a novel therapy exists that could save her life or dramatically improve her quality of life. However, the cost is insurmountable, and access is limited to specialized urban centers equipped to administer such treatments.

How do we ensure that this child has the same chance at life-saving care as one born into privilege? How do we balance incentivizing innovation with providing equitable access?

Innovative payment models known as value-based contracts are emerging to link costs to real-world outcomes. Instead of paying upfront for a miracle cure, insurers can agree to a payment plan based on the therapy's results. Value-based contracts are becoming an important strategy that links payments to real-world outcomes. These agreements often include performance metrics such as improved mobility, survival rates, specific timeframes for measurement, and potential rebates if the therapy does not meet the agreed-upon benchmarks.

Novartis' Zolgensma, a $2.1 million one-time treatment for spinal muscular atrophy, exemplifies this approach. Spinal muscular atrophy is a severe condition affecting infants, often leading to death within two years if untreated. Novartis implemented an outcomes-based payment model, allowing insurers to spread payments over five years with refund options. By 2024, this model had significantly improved access, with coverage rates reaching 90% for commercially insured patients and 30% for Medicaid patients in the U.S.

Bluebird Bio's Zynteglo for beta-thalassemia offers another example. The company guarantees an 80% reimbursement if patients don't achieve lasting benefits from the treatment, protecting payers from financial risk and incentivizing durable cures. This model protects payers from financial risk and incentivizes pharmaceutical companies to focus on delivering durable cures rather than short-term fixes.

Implementing value-based care models in healthcare presents complex and multifaceted challenges. For instance, effectively monitoring a patient's health progress over time requires consistent patient engagement and careful collection and analysis of data from various healthcare systems, each with its own protocols and metrics. A major challenge is creating a unified definition of "success," which can vary significantly depending on the specific medical condition and each patient's circumstances.

As we look to the future, medical technology is set to undergo rapid evolution, with the number of available gene therapies expected to rise by 2030. Given this promising outlook in gene therapies, finding a balance between promoting innovation and ensuring equitable access to these treatments is crucial. Improving value-based contract models is essential for achieving this goal, as it will help align incentives among providers, payers, and patients. In turn, this will enhance the overall quality and accessibility of healthcare.

While value-based contracts help reduce risks for individual payers, broader systemic solutions are needed to address the financial challenges associated with gene therapies. One promising approach is risk pooling, which involves sharing costs among large groups through insurance or government programs. This method is becoming increasingly popular to make these therapies more affordable.

Medicaid's Cell and Gene Therapy Access Model is a pioneering initiative that seeks to establish negotiated bulk pricing agreements with pharmaceutical manufacturers, all while prioritizing equitable access for underserved populations. This program is designed to purchase treatments in large quantities, which can significantly reduce costs. A key aspect of this model is its commitment to ensuring that marginalized groups, such as low-income individuals, rural communities, and those who face systemic barriers to healthcare, can access these vital therapies without encountering prohibitive financial hurdles.

In addition, the healthcare landscape is witnessing a shift towards international collaboration and enhanced manufacturing efficiencies. These are becoming increasingly vital in seeking affordable and scalable therapies accessible to patients globally.

The COVID-19 pandemic underscored the effectiveness of cross-border partnerships in expediting vaccine development and distribution. The COVAX initiative demonstrated how pooling resources, sharing expertise, and leveraging existing infrastructure enabled countries to deliver billions of vaccine doses in record time. By the end of 2021, COVAX aimed to secure and distribute two billion vaccine doses, particularly to low and middle-income countries.

The initiative initially aimed to secure and distribute two billion vaccine doses by the end of 2021. Still, it did not fully achieve this goal. COVAX reached the milestone of delivering one billion doses on January 15, 2022, slightly later than planned.

Inspired by this collaborative spirit, the gene therapy sector could benefit immensely from a similar paradigm. International alliances could pave the way for developing cost-effective generic versions of innovative therapies, ensuring they are within reach for diverse populations. Some programs are starting to pop up that capitalize on this inspiration.

The FDA launched the CoGenT Global Pilot Program in January 2024 to enhance the international regulation of gene therapies for rare diseases. This initiative promotes collaboration between regulatory agencies and encourages the harmonization of manufacturing protocols.

It builds on the success of initiatives like the Oncology Center for Excellence's Project Orbis, which facilitates concurrent international reviews of oncology products. By leveraging global patient populations and consolidating resources, CoGenT Global aims to make gene therapies more accessible and affordable worldwide.

Moreover, establishing regional manufacturing hubs could facilitate large-scale production of these treatments, addressing local needs and global health challenges. For example, New York's BioGenesis Park, a $430 million cell and gene therapy innovation hub, aims to create a robust, interconnected network that leverages complementary resources and capabilities. Such coordinated efforts could change the availability of gene therapies, ultimately enhancing health equity and health outcomes worldwide.

Companies like Orgenesis are pioneering models by placing container-sized manufacturing facilities near medical centers within a four-hour radius. Collaborations like the one between Ori Biotech and Fresenius Kabi are advancing the manufacturing of cell and gene therapies. These partnerships are designed to reduce obstacles and promote the quicker and more efficient introduction of these therapies to the market. Additionally, in May 2023, Labcorp and Forge Biologics announced a collaboration on gene therapy development and manufacturing to accelerate clinical timelines and address potential regulatory challenges.

These coordinated efforts are changing the availability of gene therapies, ultimately enhancing health equity and health outcomes worldwide. The global cell and gene therapy manufacturing market is projected to reach $10 billion by 2032, driven by the growing incidence of genetic disorders and chronic illnesses.

It is estimated that approximately one million Americans will have benefited from gene therapy treatments by the year 2034. Annual spending on gene therapies is projected to rise dramatically to about $25 billion by 2026, driven by the complexity of these treatments and the increasing number of patients seeking them. After this peak, expenditures are expected to stabilize at around $21 billion each year, leading to a more sustainable financial landscape for the industry.

These figures highlight the growing availability of gene therapies and an urgent challenge: making these life-changing treatments more affordable and accessible to patients. As the industry evolves, improving value-based contract models and exploring systemic solutions, such as risk pooling, will be essential to balance innovation with equitable access and healthcare system sustainability.

~∘

Ensuring equitable access to genetic medicine requires a coordinated effort to reduce development costs, streamline regulatory processes, and build sustainable funding models. Effective collaboration, an intricate network of partnerships among governments, pharmaceutical companies, healthcare providers, patient advocacy groups, and communities, is essential to achieving these goals.

Public-private partnerships have emerged as a pivotal force driving advancements in gene therapy, showcasing the power of collaboration between government entities and industry experts. These synergistic alliances accelerate the development and delivery of innovative treatments and tackle significant barriers to patient access. A noteworthy example of this collaboration is the Bespoke Gene Therapy Consortium, an initiative led by the Foundation for the National Institutes of Health.

With an impressive funding pool of $100 million, the Bespoke Gene Therapy Consortium brings together a vast network of 33 organizations, including prominent National Institutes of Health centers, the FDA, leading biopharmaceutical companies, and dedicated nonprofit organizations. This diverse coalition is committed to streamlining the development processes for gene therapies, especially those targeting rare diseases frequently overlooked by traditional market interests.

The Bespoke Gene Therapy Consortium has made progress by developing comprehensive, open-source playbooks that guide the manufacturing and preclinical testing phases of gene therapy. These resources help mitigate inefficiencies and expedite the journey from scientific discovery to clinical trials, ultimately making cutting-edge therapies more accessible and affordable for the patients who need them most.

Collaboration extends beyond merely pooling resources; it encompasses a shared commitment to overcoming challenges. The AcCELLerate Forum is a prime example of this collaborative spirit, uniting a diverse coalition of stakeholders, including healthcare providers, payers, government agencies, and industry leaders. Together, they are working to tackle the complex delivery challenges associated with systemic cell and gene therapies.

A pivotal area of focus for the forum is developing sustainable funding models for high-cost therapies. The price of gene therapies extends beyond the immense dollar costs. Patients are often required to navigate lengthy treatment processes, collaborating with hematologists and transplant specialists. Alongside the direct costs of these therapies, patients face additional financial strains, including lost wages due to time away from work and travel expenses to reach specialized treatment centers.

The dedicated efforts of the AcCELLerate Forum highlight the importance of collaboration in addressing the issue of exorbitant drug pricing and the often-overlooked hidden costs intrinsic to the treatment journey. By prioritizing inclusive dialogue and shared responsibility, the forum aims to create a more equitable healthcare landscape that significantly improves access to vital therapies for marginalized communities.

The future of gene therapy depends on breaking down silos between stakeholders. Researchers working in isolation must connect with policymakers shaping regulations; pharmaceutical companies must listen to patient advocates; and communities must feel empowered to participate without fear or mistrust. This need for unity is particularly evident in global health contexts.

For example, sickle cell disease affects 120 million worldwide, with 66% of cases occurring in sub-Saharan Africa. Approximately 1,000 babies are born daily in Africa with a high risk of sickle cell disease. Yet access to approved gene therapies remains almost nonexistent in low-resource settings due to prohibitive costs and inadequate healthcare infrastructure.

Organizations like the World Health Organization and the World Economic Foundation are beginning to address these disparities by promoting universal health coverage models that pool resources from government programs to finance expensive treatments for underserved populations.

However, collaboration alone cannot solve these challenges. To truly unlock the potential of gene therapy, we must build trust—

trust in science, trust in healthcare systems, and trust between stakeholders. This trust begins with education.

~✎

For many, terms like CRISPR or tandem mass spectrometry evoke the vibrant yet distant realms of science fiction, where imagination reigns and the boundaries of possibility seem limitless. Once confined to the pages of futuristic tales, these concepts might feel like distant galaxies; fascinating yet irrelevant to our daily lives. Yet these tools hold the power to transform medicine, save lives, prevent diseases, and reshape the future of healthcare.

The challenge lies not in science but in bridging the significant knowledge gap between these technologies and the general public. At the same time, building trust in genetic medicine is crucial, especially in an environment where mistrust in medical systems is a significant barrier to acceptance and understanding.

Mistrust in medicine is not a new phenomenon; it is deeply rooted in a history of systemic abuses and inequities that continue to harm marginalized communities. These historical wrongs are not merely shadows of the past. They are living legacies that shape how many people perceive and interact with healthcare systems today.

Take, for example, the infamous Tuskegee syphilis study, in which African American men were deliberately denied treatment for syphilis over four decades while being misled into believing they were receiving medical care. This allowed the disease to ravage their bodies unchecked, leaving a legacy of betrayal that continues to haunt public health efforts. Similarly, the unconsented use of Henrietta Lacks' cells, which were immortalized for their scientific contributions, exemplifies a profound violation of trust. Her genetic material was used without her knowledge or approval, raising ethical concerns that still resonate today.

These events are not just historical footnotes but enduring reminders of injustice. They have created a pervasive barrier to trust that many individuals carry into modern healthcare settings, influencing their willingness to seek treatment or participate in medical research. Modern surveys show that 57% of Black Americans remain skeptical of medical research due to historical abuses.

The tragic case of Jesse Gelsinger serves as a more modern and stark reminder of what happens when trust is betrayed in genetic research. What began as a beacon of hope spiraled into a devastating nightmare, culminating in his untimely death and casting a long shadow over the future of genetic medicine.

Jesse's death halted progress for years and left an indelible mark on public trust. Even as safety protocols have improved since Jesse's passing, subsequent cases reveal that genetic medicine remains fraught with challenges and risks. CAR-T cell therapy, a treatment for certain blood cancers such as leukemia and lymphoma, has saved countless lives by reprogramming patients' immune cells to target and attack cancer. However, this approach has also exposed the unpredictable complexities of interventions.

Between 2017 and 2023, the FDA documented 22 cases of secondary T-cell cancers following CAR-T therapy for relapsed or refractory blood cancers. In one particularly tragic case at Stanford Health Care, a patient developed fatal T-cell lymphoma just months after receiving CAR-T treatment. Molecular analyses revealed that while the CAR-T cells were not directly responsible for causing the new malignancy, the therapy weakened the patient's immune defenses, allowing pre-existing cancerous cells to thrive unchecked.

A broader study at Stanford involving 724 patients found that approximately 6.5% developed secondary blood cancers within three years of undergoing CAR-T treatment. While it is emphasized that this risk is low compared to the therapy's life-saving benefits, these cases underscore the inherent unpredictability of genetic medicine and highlight why transparency about potential risks is critical for informed consent and public trust.

The risks associated with genetic medicine extend beyond CAR-T therapies, including clinical trials targeting severe blood disorders such as beta-thalassemia and sickle cell disease. These conditions disproportionately affect marginalized communities. Some participants developed leukemia linked to viral delivery vectors used in the treatment.

One notable case involved lentiviral-based gene therapies to correct mutations causing these disorders. While these therapies significantly alleviated symptoms and improved the quality of life for many patients, some faced devastating side effects due to "insertional mutagenesis." This occurs when viral vectors integrate into patients' genomes in ways that disrupt nearby genes regulating cell growth, triggering uncontrolled proliferation and leukemia.

More recently, in the spring of 2025, it was announced that a 16-year-old patient with Duchenne muscular dystrophy tragically passed away after receiving Sarepta Therapeutics' gene therapy, Elevidys. This incident marks the first reported fatality associated with this treatment. It has renewed scrutiny of gene therapy's challenges and risks.

Elevidys, approved by the FDA for patients aged four and older with Duchenne muscular dystrophy, uses an adeno-associated virus vector to deliver a modified gene that produces microdystrophin, a shortened version of the dystrophin protein missing in patients. While this approach has shown promise in treating this devastating disease, it also carries known risks, particularly to the liver.

The patient, who received the treatment in December 2024, developed acute liver failure several months later. This severe complication led to his untimely death, despite Elevidys having been administered to over 800 individuals in clinical trials and real-world settings without previous fatalities. The case highlights the unpredictable nature of gene therapies and the potential for rare but serious adverse events.

Scientifically, liver failure likely results from a complex interplay of factors. Gene therapies using adeno-associated virus vectors can potentially cause liver damage due to the body's immune response to the viral vector. In this case, tests revealed that the patient had a recent cytomegalovirus infection, which may have contributed to the liver failure by further compromising the organ's function. The combination of gene therapy and the viral infection may have overwhelmed the patient's liver, leading to acute failure.

These stories, from Jesse Gelsinger's tragic trial outcomes to secondary cancers, underscore one unassailable truth: transparency is not optional; it is essential.

Still, rebuilding trust requires more than transparency.

Education plays a critical role in restoring confidence in genetic medicine as the field advances at an unprecedented pace. Many people remain wary of these innovations; not because they doubt their potential but because they don't fully understand them or fear how their genetic information might be misused.

Public awareness campaigns have already proven their value in demystifying complex scientific concepts and encouraging participation in genetic testing. The Genetic Cardiomyopathy Awareness Campaign, launched in 2023, highlighted the underpinnings of cardiomyopathy. In this condition, the heart muscle weakens and struggles to pump blood effectively.

Approximately 50% of cardiomyopathy cases are linked to genetic causes, yet only 1% of patients undergo testing. By raising awareness and encouraging testing among patients and their families, we can help identify individuals at risk of sudden cardiac death while advancing research into targeted therapies.

These campaigns are not just about raising awareness but about creating actionable change. They connect patients with resources, encourage family screenings, and support researchers in gathering the data needed to develop new therapies. The ripple effects are profound: lives are saved, families are empowered, and science is advanced.

Accessible tools like user-friendly apps, interactive websites, and visual aids are essential for empowering individuals to understand their genetic risks. Armed with knowledge, people can make choices that could save their lives. This is the promise of education: *turning information into empowerment.*

Real-world examples underscore this potential. In South Florida's Genetics Awareness Project, tailored educational sessions reached over 1,200 people in Black and Hispanic communities, groups often underrepresented in genetic research. The project didn't just educate. It built trust by addressing community concerns about privacy and data misuse while connecting participants with genetic counseling and testing resources.

Similarly, the Dilated Cardiomyopathy Foundation's outreach efforts for dilated cardiomyopathy have provided critical support for patients navigating their diagnoses. These programs have transformed fear into action by offering step-by-step guidance on genetic counseling and connecting families with advanced care centers specializing in heart failure.

Patient advocacy groups amplify these efforts by ensuring that therapies address real-world needs rather than abstract goals. Organizations like CureDuchenne and Parent Project Muscular Dystrophy have directly influenced clinical trial design by highlighting what matters most to patients: improvements in quality of life or minimizing side effects. Their involvement ensures that trials are not only scientifically rigorous but also patient-centered.

Education is more than just a tool; it's a vital lifeline for advancing genetic medicine in an equitable and ethical manner. By simplifying complex concepts through public awareness campaigns, providing accessible resources tailored to various communities, and amplifying patient voices through advocacy groups, we can bridge the knowledge gap that currently hinders progress. However, education alone is insufficient; additional systemic efforts and considerations are also needed.

As collaboration, education, and trust accelerate progress in genetic medicine, ethical frameworks must evolve just as rapidly. The expansion of screening and therapies forces us to confront questions about privacy, data security, and consent—questions at the heart of whether genetic medicine can fulfill its promise equitably and ethically.

Who owns genetic data? How do we protect sensitive information while fostering collaboration? And how do we balance an individual's right to privacy with their family's right to know about shared genetic risks?

These are not abstract dilemmas; they are pressing, real-world challenges. Genetic data is profoundly personal yet inherently shared. It reveals intimate details about an individual's health, ancestry, and predispositions while offering insights into their family and broader community.

This interconnectedness is both a strength and a challenge. On one hand, it enables us to uncover patterns that lead to breakthroughs in understanding diseases like cancer or heart disease. Conversely, it raises ethical dilemmas about consent, ownership, and responsibility.

Take the case of Kathleen Folbigg. Convicted in 2003 for the deaths of her four children, Folbigg was exonerated in 2023 after genomic evidence revealed that her daughters carried a rare mutation linked to sudden cardiac death. Sequencing her genome didn't just rewrite her story; it reshaped her family's medical history. While this knowledge clarified one family's tragedy, it also exposed sensitive information about relatives who may share similar mutations.

Such cases force us to ask: *Who has the right to know about shared risks? Conversely, who has the right **not** to know?*

217

These questions are not hypothetical. They play out in real-world scenarios. In 1977, Jim and Barbara Pryce were expecting twins, Kim and Kelly, when they received a call from a doctor who had diagnosed Jim's mother with Huntington's disease. The doctor warned Jim that he and other family members might be at risk. Jim received genetic counseling, and initial tests were inconclusive but seemed reassuring.

Initial tests seemed reassuring, but the specter of the disease never truly faded. Huntington's disease is a single mutation with the power to alter lives irrevocably. For the children of those affected, there is a 50% chance of inheriting the gene that will almost certainly lead to the disease.

Fifteen years later, Barbara and the children began to notice changes in Jim. Kim recalls that her father seemed stressed and more irritable than usual, and she noticed shaking movements in his hands, similar to those of her grandmother. By this time, the Pryce family included two more daughters, Tracy and Erin. As Jim's symptoms progressed, the family pulled together to care for him, with Barbara taking on the primary caregiving role.

For Jim, the disease stole not just his health but his identity. Jim's illness took a toll on his career. A physical therapist, like Barbara, he was forced to stop practicing. A fall in 2000 accelerated his decline, impacting his balance and dexterity.

As the sisters entered adulthood, they faced a choice that would shape the rest of their lives: whether to undergo genetic testing for Huntington's. Kimberly first broached the subject in 2003, her desire to start a family pushing her to confront the unknown. She described the testing process as a flip of a coin. Heads, you are facing a progressive and life-threatening brain disease that you can pass on to your children. Tails, you are okay.

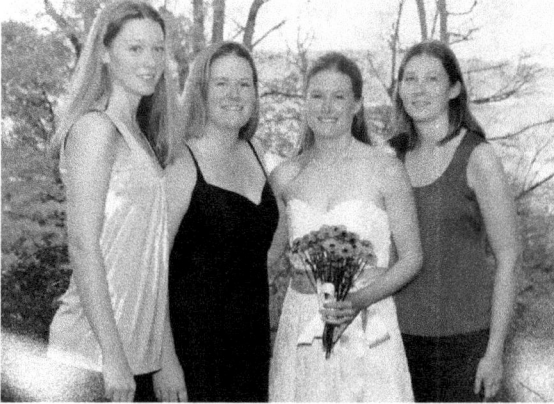

Figure 63. The Pryce Sisters. The Johns Hopkins University

One by one, the sisters made their choice. The twins, Kim and Kelly, were tested first, and their results returned negative. Tracy was also tested and received a negative result, and soon became pregnant. For Erin, the youngest, the test was positive, confirming that she carried the Huntington's gene. The news hit the family like a thunderbolt, each sister grappling with a complex mix of emotions. Relief, guilt, fear, and determination swirled together, binding them even closer in the face of this shared challenge.

Erin, rather than retreating into despair, chose to face her diagnosis head-on. She chose to be open about her diagnosis, becoming a fierce advocate for Huntington's research and awareness. She actively raises funds for the Huntington's Disease Society of America and participates in research studies.

"The disease didn't end for our family when we lost my grandmother, and it didn't end with my father," she declared. "But it will end with me."

The Pryce family's story vividly illustrates the complex ethical landscape of genetic medicine, particularly regarding the right to know and the right not to know about shared risks. As Erin Pryce declared her determination to end Huntington's disease in her family, her story opened up a broader discussion on the ethical implications of genetic testing and information sharing.

The decision-making process the Pryce sisters went through, choosing whether to undergo testing for Huntington's disease, highlights the profound personal and familial implications of genetic information. Their experience raises critical questions about consent, privacy, and the responsibility to share potentially life-altering information with family members.

These questions are not merely theoretical but have real-world consequences. As medicine advances, the ethical frameworks governing its use must evolve to address the unique challenges posed by the familial nature of genetic data. The interconnectedness of gene information means that one person's decision to undergo testing can have far-reaching implications for their living and unborn relatives.

Who has the right to know about shared genetic risks? If you inherited the gene, should you also "inherit" the data about that gene?

This question becomes particularly poignant when considering scenarios where one family member's genetic test results could provide crucial health information to others. The European Court of Human Rights has recognized that the capacity of data to identify relationships between individuals is sufficient to constitute a serious interference with the right to private life. This recognition underscores the need for a more nuanced approach to genetic privacy that considers the interests of biological relatives.

Conversely, the right not to know is equally complex. Some individuals may prefer not to know their predispositions, especially for conditions like Huntington's disease, for which there is currently no cure. *How do we balance this preference against the potential benefits of early intervention or lifestyle changes that could mitigate risks?*

The case of the Pryce family also highlights the importance of genetic counseling and informed consent. As genetic testing becomes more widespread, healthcare providers must ensure that individuals understand the personal implications of their test results and the potential impact on their family members. This understanding is crucial for making informed decisions about testing and sharing results.

Furthermore, the Pryce sisters' story underscores the need for clear guidelines on when and how healthcare providers can disclose genetic information to at-risk relatives, especially in cases where the tested individual refuses to share the information. Balancing the duty of confidentiality with the potential to prevent harm to others remains a challenging ethical dilemma in genetic medicine.

As we move forward, it is clear that the success of genetic medicine depends on creating systems that can effectively connect researchers, healthcare providers, and patients while safeguarding privacy. These systems are not mere logistical necessities; they are lifelines for patients navigating the complexities of genetic medicine. However, creating them requires balancing two often competing priorities: the need for broad data sharing to advance science and the need to protect individual privacy.

Consider platforms like the National Institutes of Health's Genomic Data Sharing initiative, which houses vast amounts of de-identified genomic data worldwide. These databases are invaluable for scientific progress, but come with risks. A 2013 study demonstrated how individuals could be re-identified by combining de-identified genomic data with genealogical databases and public records. This vulnerability underscores the limitations of anonymization in genomics. DNA is unique and permanent, unlike other health data, making true anonymity nearly impossible.

To address these risks, the National Institutes of Health controls access to sensitive information through strict protocols. Similarly, the UK Biobank, one of the largest genomic databases globally, has implemented robust safeguards prohibiting identifying participants or using data for non-research purposes like law enforcement or insurance decisions. Yet even with these protections in place, concerns persist about how genomic data might be used in ways participants never anticipated.

Direct-to-consumer genetic testing companies like 23andMe further complicate matters. As we discussed earlier, these companies have suffered tremendous data breaches. More recently, there has been contention about what the company's bankruptcy means for those with their genetic data in 23andMe's database.

Despite assurances from 23andMe, experts fear that the company's assets, including amassed DNA data, could fall into the wrong hands during the sale process. The Office of California's Attorney General and the UK's Information Commissioner's Office have issued warnings, advising customers to delete their data and emphasizing strict data protection standards. This situation highlights the potential for misuse of data and the importance of robust security measures and transparent data handling practices in the genetic testing industry.

In a notable case involving Vitagene, now known as 1Health, sensitive data was unintentionally exposed on a publicly accessible, unsecured cloud server. Over 2,000 clients had their personal information, including health reports and raw genetic data, in easily accessible cloud "buckets." The company received warnings thrice over two years regarding the risks of storing unencrypted data in publicly accessible locations.

As a result, the company was fined $75,000 for misleading consumers about its data-sharing practices and for failing to protect their privacy. The company was also required to issue refunds to affected customers and is now subject to increased scrutiny from the Federal Trade Commission. This breach underscored how lax security practices can erode trust.

Many consumers are unaware that agreeing to the terms of service, typically hidden in the fine print, permits companies to use their genetic information for research or commercial purposes. For example, 23andMe partnered with Calico, a Google spinoff, giving them access to its databases for longevity research. Additionally, GlaxoSmithKline announced plans to use 23andMe's databases to identify pharmaceutical targets.

One of the most contentious issues in genetic medicine is ownership of data. In the United States, laws like HIPAA provide some protections for medical information, but do not explicitly address who owns genomic data once it is collected. Some states have begun to frame genetic material as an individual's property.

For example, Alaska passed legislation declaring DNA samples as the *"exclusive property"* of the person they were collected. However, this approach remains inconsistent across jurisdictions.

In contrast, European regulations grant individuals explicit control over their data, including genomic information. These protections ensure that individuals must provide informed consent before their data can be used and that they retain the right to withdraw consent at any time.

Navigating these challenges requires robust ethical oversight and legal protections tailored to the unique nature of genomic data. Platforms like Concert Genetics' proposed "Genetic Health Information Network" envision a future where patients can securely share genomic data with authorized providers across healthcare systems. Such interoperability could eliminate care gaps for underserved populations while ensuring consistent access to cutting-edge treatments.

The World Health Organization's recently released principles for ethical human genomic data collection and sharing represent a pivotal step toward addressing the complex challenges surrounding privacy, equity, and responsible data use in genetic medicine. These guidelines emphasize transparency, informed consent, and equity to ensure that genomic advancements benefit diverse populations without reinforcing health disparities.

However, while these principles provide a critical ethical foundation, the practical delivery of genetic medicine remains fragmented and inconsistent. Bridging this gap requires robust ethical frameworks and standardized care protocols to ensure that therapies reach patients equitably and effectively.

～𝇋

Currently, the delivery of genetic medicine is far from seamless. Guidelines for managing gene-based conditions change frequently, making it challenging for healthcare providers to stay up to date. This lack of consistency creates significant barriers for patients, who risk receiving outdated or incomplete advice about their genetic risks and treatment options. Without standardized protocols, the promise of gene medicine can falter at the point of care.

Take hereditary cancer syndromes as an example. For individuals carrying BRCA1 or BRCA2 mutations, clear guidelines linking screening results to actionable steps, such as increased surveillance or preventive surgeries, can mean the difference between early detection and late-stage diagnoses.

Programs like Helix's health system partnerships illustrate how integrating screening results directly into patient medical records can transform genetic testing from a passive exercise into a proactive tool for disease prevention. These systems empower patients and providers by ensuring that follow-up care is automatic rather than optional.

Standardized care protocols are essential for improving patient outcomes and addressing disparities in access to genetic medicine. Care delivery can vary widely without clear guidelines depending on geography, institutional resources, or individual provider expertise. This inconsistency disproportionately impacts underserved populations, who are already less likely to have access to cutting-edge treatments.

For example, in rural areas where specialist care is limited, patients with hereditary conditions may not receive the same level of surveillance as those in urban centers with dedicated genetic counseling teams. Standardized protocols could help bridge this gap by providing clear, evidence-based recommendations that any healthcare provider can follow, regardless of location.

The ethical principles outlined by the WHO must also be embedded into the practical delivery of genetic medicine. Transparency and informed consent are foundational to building trust between patients and providers. However, these principles must extend beyond data collection to encompass every stage of care delivery.

Consider secondary findings: unexpected results uncovered during genetic testing that may reveal risks unrelated to the original reason for testing. For instance, a patient undergoing testing for cardiomyopathy might inadvertently learn they carry a mutation linked to Alzheimer's disease or another unrelated condition. Current gaps allow secondary uses of genomic data without explicit consent, a loophole undermining trust in medical research.

How should these findings be communicated? What responsibilities do healthcare providers have to inform patients—or their families—of these risks?

The future of medicine depends on our ability to merge ethical principles with practical delivery systems. Strengthening laws around genetic privacy is a critical first step.

~9

As efforts to standardize care protocols in genetic medicine advance, it becomes increasingly clear that public awareness and systemic improvements alone are insufficient. The success of gene medicine depends significantly on healthcare professionals who interpret complex genetic data and guide patients through life-altering decisions. However, many providers lack the specialized training to navigate this rapidly evolving field.

To address this gap, it is essential to integrate genomics into medical training programs worldwide, ensuring that specialists and all healthcare providers who interact with patients are adequately prepared. Genetic medicine is advancing breathtakingly, but many healthcare providers struggle to keep up. The sheer volume of discoveries, ranging from gene therapies to pharmacogenomics, requires a level of expertise that most medical professionals were not trained for during their education.

This knowledge gap has real consequences. A survey revealed that only 20% of physicians felt confident in interpreting genetic test results. Also, 41% of physicians indicated that insufficient training in identifying appropriate tests and analyzing the results was the most significant barrier to ordering tests for their patients.

Another study surveyed 123 physicians regarding their familiarity with genetic tests. While 38% of the participants felt confident in their knowledge, only 6% achieved a high score in the knowledge assessment. Notably, one-third of the physicians had never ordered testing, primarily due to their lack of knowledge. Without proper training, even well-meaning providers may inadvertently misinterpret results, leading to unnecessary anxiety or missed opportunities for early intervention.

Integrating genomics into medical education is essential to ensuring that all providers can effectively guide patients through the complexities of medicine. Initiatives like Medical Genetics Awareness Week, organized by the American College of Medical

Genetics and Genomics, are beginning to address this need. This annual event celebrates the contributions of medical genetics teams while educating other healthcare professionals about their role in patient care.

During Medical Genetics Awareness Week, participants gain access to resources such as toolkits, webinars, and mentorship opportunities designed to demystify genetics for non-specialists. For example, a recent session focused on how primary care physicians can incorporate pharmacogenomics into routine practice, enabling them to prescribe medications tailored to a patient's genetic profile. These efforts aim to empower providers with the knowledge and confidence to integrate genetics into everyday clinical decision-making.

Programs like Helix's partnerships with major health systems demonstrate how training can transform care delivery. Helix has helped train thousands of providers to interpret genomic data effectively by collaborating with institutions like Sanford Health and HealthPartners. These partnerships include hands-on workshops where clinicians learn how to integrate insights into electronic health records and use them for early detection and prevention of diseases like breast cancer or high cholesterol.

For instance, Sanford Health's population genomics initiative has enrolled over 100,000 participants in a DNA testing program to identify individuals at risk for inherited conditions. Providers working within this system receive ongoing training on interpreting test results and communicating findings to patients in clear and actionable ways. This approach improves patient outcomes and fosters greater trust between providers and their communities.

Technology is increasingly vital in equipping healthcare professionals with the tools they need to succeed in genetic medicine. Platforms like PharmGKB and ClinVar provide centralized databases where providers can access up-to-date information about pharmacogenetic alleles and variants. These resources simplify translating complex genomic data into actionable insights to improve patient care.

Similarly, electronic health records are being adapted to include decision-support tools that guide providers in interpreting genetic information at the point of care. For example, a clinician prescribing medication for a patient with a known variant affecting drug metabolism might receive an automated alert recommending an alternative treatment. By embedding these tools directly into clinical workflows, technology helps bridge the gap between genomic research and real-world application.

Preparing healthcare professionals for the future of genetic medicine requires more than one-off training sessions; it demands a systemic change in how medical education is structured. Medical and nursing schools and residency programs must begin incorporating genomics into their curricula as a core competency rather than an optional specialization.

Some institutions are already leading the way. The University of California, San Francisco, recently launched a pilot program where medical students complete clinical rotations alongside genetic counselors and researchers in precision medicine clinics. This immersive experience allows future physicians to see firsthand how genetics can inform diagnosis and treatment across specialties.

In addition to formal education, continuing medical education programs are critical for keeping practicing clinicians up-to-date.

Organizations like the Clinical Pharmacogenetics Implementation Consortium offer courses integrating pharmacogenomics into routine practice. These courses provide practical guidance on ordering genetic tests, interpreting results, and discussing findings with patients.

When healthcare providers are well-trained in genetics, the benefits extend beyond individual patients. They ripple outward throughout communities. A provider who understands how to interpret BRCA1 test results can help their patients and their family members who may share similar risks. Similarly, a primary care physician trained in pharmacogenomics can prevent adverse drug reactions by tailoring prescriptions based on genetic profiles.

This ripple effect is significant for addressing disparities in access to genetic medicine. In rural or underserved areas with limited access to specialists, well-trained primary care providers can be critical links between patients and cutting-edge treatments.

Integrating genomics into routine healthcare represents one of the most significant shifts in modern medicine, but it cannot succeed without a workforce equipped to navigate its complexities. Training programs must be expanded and standardized across institutions, ensuring every provider has the tools to deliver personalized care.

The future of gene therapy is not some distant horizon—it is here, unfolding one breakthrough at a time. In 2024 alone, CRISPR-based therapies reached their first commercial applications, offering curative treatments for conditions like sickle cell disease and beta-thalassemia.

Advances in manufacturing efficiency are making once-unimaginable therapies more scalable. Clinical trials are expanding into new areas, from autoimmune diseases to solid tumors. The momentum is undeniable. Gene therapy is no longer a promise; it is a reality that is reshaping medicine and rewriting the possibilities of human health.

But the true power of this revolution lies not just in science, but in its impact on people. You may recall from earlier in this book that the Villarreal family endured a parent's worst nightmare as they confronted the heartbreaking diagnosis of spinal muscular atrophy type 1 in their baby daughter, Evelyn. Spinal muscular atrophy gradually paralyzes infants, stripping them of their ability to move, breathe, and ultimately, survive past the age of two. The family is deeply aware of this as their first daughter, Josephine, lost her battle with the disease at only 15 months old.

When Evelyn was born, joy quickly turned to dread as genetic testing confirmed she, too, had spinal muscular atrophy. Milan recalled thinking, "We knew what we were dealing with: We'll love her for as long as we can."

That same night, driven by desperation and a glimmer of hope, they urgently searched the internet and discovered a clinical trial in Ohio. At just eight weeks old, Evelyn became one of the first babies to receive Zolgensma. Today, Evelyn is a bubbly, red-haired toddler who defies all expectations. While she has some weakness in her thighs and can't run or jump like other children, she can walk quickly, dance, trace letters, carry a chair, and climb onto her mother's lap. Every milestone, every step forward, was a moment of profound joy and celebration for the Villarreals.

These stories are anecdotes and testaments to what is possible when innovation meets compassion. They remind us that behind every clinical trial, every data point, and every regulatory approval is a person with a name, a story, and a future that genetic medicine has the power to transform.

We must embrace possibilities while acknowledging challenges. These challenges also highlight what must be done: we must prioritize honesty about risks as much as we celebrate breakthroughs. Transparency builds trust, which is the foundation upon which all progress rests. Without it, even the most innovative therapies will fail to reach those who need them most.

This is not just about science—it is about humanity. It is about families who dared to hope when all seemed lost, patients who turned fear into action, communities that found empowerment through education, and even those grappling with difficult ethical questions about shared genetic risks.

It is also about you, the reader, who now understands that *this revolution belongs to all of us.* Whether as patients, advocates, researchers, or simply members of society, we each have a role to play in shaping this future responsibly.

We stand at the precipice of a new era, where the blueprint of our lives is no longer an immutable script but a text we can edit, refine, and, in some cases, rewrite entirely. Once a game of chance dictated health and fate, the gene pool is now subject to our intervention. The knowledge we've gleaned, unraveling the double helix, deciphering the code, and now wielding the tools to alter it, has propelled us from passive observers to active authors of our genetic narrative.

232

Envision a future where the specter of hereditary diseases fades away, as proactive gene edits serve as a potent armor against genetic predispositions. Picture a world where a single transformative treatment can free individuals from lifelong afflictions. This is a reality where the whims of fate in our birth no longer dictate our destinies.

Yet, the power to rewrite destiny carries profound responsibility. *How do we ensure equitable access to these life-altering therapies? How do we balance the pursuit of innovation with the imperative of ethical stewardship? How do we build trust in systems that have, in the past, betrayed that very trust?*

These are not abstract policy questions but human dilemmas that demand our collective attention. The answers will not be found in scientific breakthroughs alone but in our choices: funding, regulation, access, and empathy. The future of genetic medicine is not predetermined. It is shaped by every decision we make, every dollar we invest, and every conversation about its promise and perils.

The ink of our genetic code is now in our hands. *Will we use it to create a future where health is a universal right, the genetic potential is unlocked for all, and the power to rewrite our genes serves humanity's highest aspirations?*

The choice, ultimately, is ours.

Dare we write a new future?

References

In this book, referencing is organized by chapter to facilitate a more streamlined and accessible reading experience. Each chapter includes its own set of references, allowing readers to easily locate sources relevant to the specific content discussed within that section.

Chapter 1

1. CDC. Real Stories About Lynch Syndrome. Hereditary Colorectal (Colon) Cancer. Published October 16, 2024. https://www.cdc.gov/colorectal-cancer-hereditary/stories/index.html

2. Domaina F : English: Autosomal dominant - genetics (english version)Français : Transmission autosomique dominante avec un parent porteur (version anglaise). Wikimedia Commons. Published March 3, 2012. https://commons.wikimedia.org/w/index.php?curid=1856701

3. O'Connor C, Miko I. Developing the Chromosome Theory | Learn Science at Scitable. Nature.com. Published 2014. https://www.nature.com/scitable/topicpage/developing-the-chromosome-theory-164/

4. Choi J, Spencer C, Kerr S, Weigel E, Montoya J. Chromosome theory of inheritance | Biological Principles.

bioprinciples.biosci.gatech.edu. Published 2023.
https://bioprinciples.biosci.gatech.edu/module-4-genes-and-genomes/4-4-linkage-sex-linkage-and-pedigree-analysis/

5. Lewis EB. The Nobel Prize in Physiology or Medicine 1933. NobelPrize.org. Published 2019.
https://www.nobelprize.org/prizes/medicine/1933/morgan/article/

6. O'connor C. Discovery of DNA as the Hereditary Material | Learn Science at Scitable. Nature.com. Published 2013.
https://www.nature.com/scitable/topicpage/discovery-of-dna-as-the-hereditary-material-340/

7. PBS. A Science Odyssey: People and Discoveries: Watson and Crick describe structure of DNA. www.pbs.org. Published 1998.
https://www.pbs.org/wgbh/aso/databank/entries/do53dn.html

8. Sutton B. The story behind Photograph 51 | Feature from King's College London. www.kcl.ac.uk. Published April 14, 2023. https://www.kcl.ac.uk/the-story-behind-photograph-51

9. Betts E. Isaac Newton Monograph.
https://edwardbetts.com/monograph/Isaac_Newton

10. WATSON JD, CRICK FHC. Molecular Structure of Nucleic Acids: A Structure for Deoxyribose Nucleic Acid. Nature. 1953;171(4356):737-738.
doi:https://doi.org/10.1038/171737a0.

11. Snider L. DNA and RNA Basics: Replication, Transcription, and Translation. www.visiblebody.com.

Published June 22, 2021.
https://www.visiblebody.com/blog/dna-and-rna-basics-replication-transcription-and-translation

12. Jack Westin. Base Pairing Specificity A With T G With C - Nucleic Acid Structure And Function - MCAT Content. Jack Westin. Published March 4, 2020. https://jackwestin.com/resources/mcat-content/nucleic-acid-structure-and-function/base-pairing-specificity-a-with-t-g-with-c

13. Thapa R. DNA Replication: Definition, Enzymes, Steps, Applications. microbenotes.com. Published August 3, 2023. https://microbenotes.com/dna-replication-steps/

14. Ghannam JY, Wang J, Jan A. Biochemistry, DNA Structure. PubMed. Published 2020. https://www.ncbi.nlm.nih.gov/books/NBK538241/

15. Bates S. Base Pair. Genome.gov. Published 2019. https://www.genome.gov/genetics-glossary/Base-Pair

16. Crick FH. General Nature of the Genetic Code for Proteins | Learn Science at Scitable. www.nature.com. Published December 30, 1961. https://www.nature.com/scitable/content/General-Nature-of-the-Genetic-Code-for-12353/

17. Hernandez V. The Debate over DNA Replication Before the Meselson-Stahl Experiment (1953–1957) | The Embryo Project Encyclopedia. Asu.edu. Published 2018. https://embryo.asu.edu/pages/debate-over-dna-replication-meselson-stahl-experiment-1953-1957

18. Meselson M, Stahl FW. 1958: Semiconservative Replication of DNA. Genome.gov. Published 1958. https://www.genome.gov/25520258/online-education-kit-1958-semiconservative-replication-of-dna.

19. Mercadante AA, Dimri M, Mohiuddin SS. Biochemistry, Replication and Transcription. PubMed. Published August 14, 2023. https://www.ncbi.nlm.nih.gov/books/NBK540152/.

20. Your Genome. How is DNA turned into protein? www.yourgenome.org. https://www.yourgenome.org/theme/how-is-dna-turned-into-protein-the-central-dogma-of-molecular-biology/.

21. ATDBIO. ATDBio - Transcription, Translation and Replication. atdbio.com. Published 2024. https://atdbio.com/nucleic-acids-book/Transcription-Translation-and-Replication

22. Hu WS ., Hughes SH. HIV-1 Reverse Transcription. Cold Spring Harbor Perspectives in Medicine. 2012;2(10):a006882-a006882. doi:https://doi.org/10.1101/cshperspect.a006882

23. NCBI. RNA Interference (RNAi). Nih.gov. Published 2017. https://www.ncbi.nlm.nih.gov/probe/docs/techrnai/

24. Bergtrom G. 11.4: Breaking the Genetic Code. Biology LibreTexts. Published May 9, 2022. https://bio.libretexts.org/Under_Construction/Cell_and_Molecular_Biology_(Bergtrom)/11:_The_Genetic_Code_and_Translation/11.04:_Breaking_the_Genetic_Code

25. National Institutes of Health. Deciphering the Genetic Code - National Historic Chemical Landmark. American Chemical Society. Published November 12, 2009. https://www.acs.org/education/whatischemistry/landmarks/geneticcode.html

26. Clancy S, Brown W. Translation: DNA to mRNA to Protein. Nature.com. Published 2008. https://www.nature.com/scitable/topicpage/translation-dna-to-mrna-to-protein-393/27.

27. CDC. Genetic Disorders. Genomics and Your Health. Published May 17, 2024. https://www.cdc.gov/genomics-and-health/about/genetic-disorders.html

Chapter 2

28. Marks L. Gene therapy. WhatisBiotechnology.org. Published 2014. https://www.whatisbiotechnology.org/index.php/science/summary/gene-therapy/

29. Scangos G, Ruddle FH. Mechanisms and applications of DNA-mediated gene transfer in mammalian cells — a review. Gene. 1981;14(1-2):1-10. doi:https://doi.org/10.1016/0378-1119(81)90143-8

30. U.S. National Library of Medicine. How does gene therapy work? MedlinePlus. Published September 17, 2020. https://medlineplus.gov/genetics/understanding/therapy/procedures/

31. Bell S, Kolobova I, Crapper L, Ernst C. Lesch-Nyhan Syndrome: Models, Theories, and Therapies. Molecular

Syndromology. 2016;7(6):302-311.
doi:https://doi.org/10.1159/000449296

32. Jinnah HA, Visser JE. History | www.Lesch-Nyhan.org.
www.lesch-nyhan.org. https://www.lesch-
nyhan.org/en/definition/history

33. National Center for Biotechnology Information (US.
Lesch-Nyhan syndrome. Nih.gov. Published 2016.
https://www.ncbi.nlm.nih.gov/books/NBK22194/

34. Eren K, Taktakoglu N, Pirim I. DNA Sequencing
Methods: From Past to Present. The Eurasian Journal of
Medicine. 2023;54(Suppl):S47-S56.
doi:https://doi.org/10.5152/eurasianjmed.2022.22280

35. Medicover Hospitals. Hyperargininemia: Symptoms and
Treatment. Medicoverhospitals.in. Published 2024.
https://www.medicoverhospitals.in/diseases/hyperargininem
ia/

36. Friedmann T. Stanfield Rogers: Insights into Virus Vectors
and Failure of an Early Gene Therapy Model. Molecular
Therapy. 2001;4(4):285-288.
doi:https://doi.org/10.1006/mthe.2001.0454

37. 37.Friedmann T, Roblin R. Gene Therapy for Human
Genetic Disease? Science. 1972;175(4025):949-955.
doi:https://doi.org/10.1126/science.175.4025.949

38. Vaghela A, Payal Jethva, Ishita Zalavadiya. A
Comprehensive Exploration of Gene Therapy and its
Transformative Applications. Journal of Advanced
Pharmacy Research. 2024;0(0).
doi:https://doi.org/10.21608/aprh.2024.267430.1252

39. Terheggen HG, Lowenthal A, Lavinha F, Colombo JP, Rogers S. Unsuccessful trial of gene replacement in arginase deficiency. European Journal of Pediatrics. 1975;119(1):1-3. doi:https://doi.org/10.1007/bf00464689

40. Bulcha JT, Wang Y, Ma H, Tai PWL, Gao G. Viral vector platforms within the gene therapy landscape. Signal Transduction and Targeted Therapy. 2021;6(1). doi:https://doi.org/10.1038/s41392-021-00487-6

41. Wadbudhe AM, Meshram RJ, Tidke SC. Severe Combined Immunodeficiency (SCID) and Its New Treatment Modalities. Cureus. 2023;15(10):e47759. doi:https://doi.org/10.7759/cureus.47759

42. Your Genome. Treating the bubble babies: gene therapy in use. www.yourgenome.org. https://www.yourgenome.org/theme/treating-the-bubble-babies-gene-therapy-in-use/

43. Földesi B. The First Human Gene Therapy. Biomol GmbH - Life Science Shop. Published 2018. https://www.biomol.com/resources/biomol-blog/the-first-human-gene-therapy

44. Philippidis A. Making History with the 1990 Gene Therapy Trial. GEN - Genetic Engineering and Biotechnology News. Published March 10, 2016. https://www.genengnews.com/insights/making-history-with-the-1990-gene-therapy-trial/

45. Donovan K, Guzman N. Ornithine Transcarbamylase Deficiency. PubMed. Published August 8, 2022. https://www.ncbi.nlm.nih.gov/books/NBK537257/

46. Sibbald B. Death but one unintended consequence of gene-therapy trial. CMAJ: Canadian Medical Association Journal. 2001;164(11):1612. https://pmc.ncbi.nlm.nih.gov/articles/PMC81135/

47. Gelsinger P. Jesse's Intent. Published 2001. http://www.circare.org/submit/jintent.pdf

48. Lehrman S. Virus treatment questioned after gene therapy death. Nature. 1999;401(6753):517-518. doi:https://doi.org/10.1038/43977

49. Wold WSM, Toth K. Adenovirus vectors for gene therapy, vaccination and cancer gene therapy. Current gene therapy. 2013;13(6):421-433. doi:https://doi.org/10.2174/1566523213666131125095046

50. Cross R. The redemption of James Wilson, gene therapy pioneer. Acs.org. Published 2022. https://cen.acs.org/business/The-redemption-of-James-Wilson-gene-therapy-pioneer/97/i36

51. BBC. BBC - Science & Nature - Horizon - Trial and Error. Bbc.co.uk. Published 2014. Accessed December 4, 2024. https://www.bbc.co.uk/science/horizon/2003/trialerrortrans.shtml

52. Gorsky K. Ghosts of Gene Therapies Past- Lessons Learned From Jesse Gelsinger. Health Science Inquiry. 2019;6(1). doi:https://doi.org/10.29173/hsi200

53. Stein R. The Gelsinger Case Background. https://www.uab.edu/ccts/images/steinbrook_Gelsinger_-_Oxford_Textbook_08_3.pdf

54. Stolberg SG. Teenager's Death Is Shaking Up Field of Human Gene-Therapy Experiments. The New York Times. https://www.nytimes.com/2000/01/27/us/teenager-s-death-is-shaking-up-field-of-human-gene-therapy-experiments.html. Published January 27, 2000.

55. Wenner M. Gene therapy: An Interview with an Unfortunate Pioneer. Scientific American. Published September 1, 2009. https://www.scientificamerican.com/article/gene-therapy-an-interview/

56. Smaglik P. Investigators Ponder What Went Wrong. The Scientist Magazine®. Published October 24, 1999. https://www.the-scientist.com/investigators-ponder-what-went-wrong-56301

57. Bioethics Today. Blog - A comment from Paul Gelsinger on gene therapy and informed consent - Bioethics Today. Bioethics Today. Published February 11, 2022. https://bioethicstoday.org/blog/a-comment-from-paul-gelsinger-on-gene-therapy-and/

58. Lenzi RN, Altevogt BM, Gostin LO, on C, Board, Institute of Medicine. Oversight of Gene Transfer Research. Nih.gov. Published March 27, 2014. https://www.ncbi.nlm.nih.gov/books/NBK195894/

59. NYU Langone Health. Gene Therapy Research & the Case of Jesse Gelsinger. NYU Langone Health. Published 2024. https://med.nyu.edu/departments-institutes/population-health/divisions-sections-centers/medical-ethics/education/high-school-bioethics-project/learning-scenarios/jesse-gelsinger-case

60. U.S. Department of Justice. 2/15/05, Gene Therapy Study - Almanac, Vol. 51, No. 21. almanac.upenn.edu. Published February 15, 2005. https://almanac.upenn.edu/archive/volumes/v51/n21/gts.html

61. Rinde M. The Death of Jesse Gelsinger, 20 Years Later. Science History Institute. Published June 4, 2019. https://www.sciencehistory.org/stories/magazine/the-death-of-jesse-gelsinger-20-years-later/

62. National Human Genome Research Institute. Human Genome Project. National Human Genome Research Institute. Published August 24, 2022. https://www.genome.gov/about-genomics/educational-resources/fact-sheets/human-genome-project

63. National Human Genome Research Institute. Human Genome Project Timeline. Genome.gov. Published July 5, 2022. https://www.genome.gov/human-genome-project/timeline

64. National Human Genome Research Institute (NHGRI). International Consortium Completes Human Genome Project All Goals Achieved; New Vision for Genome Research Unveiled. Published 2003. https://www.genome.gov/11006929/2003-release-international-consortium-completes-hgp

65. HudsonAlpha. The Human Genome Project: Thirty years later – HudsonAlpha Institute for Biotechnology. https://www.hudsonalpha.org/the-human-genome-project-thirty-years-later/

66. My Lifelong Fight Against Disease - Amplify Publishing Group. Amplify Publishing Group. Published October 20, 2023. https://amplifypublishinggroup.com/product/nonfiction/health-medicine-and-wellness/general-health-medicine-and-wellness/my-lifelong-fight-against-disease-from-polio-and-aids-to-covid-19/

67. HUMAN GENOME SCIENCES. HUMAN GENOME SCIENCES ISSUED THREE U.S. HUMAN GENE PATENTS. Archive.org. Published 1996. https://web.archive.org/web/20060311080157/http://www.hgsi.com/news/press/96-04-16_patents.html

68. Human Genome Sciences. Press Release - July 16, 1996. Archive.org. Published 2024. https://web.archive.org/web/20060311080140/http://www.hgsi.com/news/press/96-07-16_Merck.html

69. McNamee LM, Ledley FD. Assessing the history and value of Human Genome Sciences. Commercialbiotechnology.com. Published 2024. Accessed December 4, 2024. https://commercialbiotechnology.com/article-detail/?id=619

70. Journal of Commercial Biotechnology. View of Assessing the history and value of Human Genome Sciences. Commercialbiotechnology.com. Published 2024. https://commercialbiotechnology.com/menuscript/index.php/jcb/article/view/619/580

71. Human Genome Sciences. Press Release - October 30, 2000. Archive.org. Published 2024.

https://web.archive.org/web/20060311074346/http://www.h
gsi.com/news/press/00-10-30_BLyS_ACR.html

72. Anderson R, Rothwell E, Botkin JR. Newborn Screening.
Annual review of nursing research. 2011;29:113-132.
doi:https://doi.org/10.1891/0739-6686.29.113

73. Halbisen AL, Lu CY. Trends in Availability of Genetic
Tests in the United States, 2012–2022. Journal of
Personalized Medicine. 2023;13(4):638.
doi:https://doi.org/10.3390/jpm13040638

74. National Human Genome Research Institute (NHGRI).
Newborn Genetic Screening. Genome.gov.
https://www.genome.gov/genetics-glossary/Newborn-
Genetic-Screening

75. Alliance G, Health D of CD of. Newborn Screening.
Genetic Alliance; 2010.
https://www.ncbi.nlm.nih.gov/books/NBK132148/

76. Dubay KS, Zach TL. Newborn Screening. PubMed.
Published 2022.
https://www.ncbi.nlm.nih.gov/books/NBK558983/

77. CDC. Little Feet Make Big Footprints in Health. Newborn
Screening. Published 2024. https://www.cdc.gov/newborn-
screening/featurestory/little-feet-big-footprints.html

78. Novartis Gene Therapies, Inc. What is spinal muscular
atrophy (SMA)? ZOLGENSMA.
https://www.zolgensma.com/about-sma

Chapter 3

79. AskanAcademic.com. How much DNA is in a human being? Ask an Academic. Published April 6, 2017. https://askanacademic.com/science/how-much-dna-is-in-a-human-being-871/

80. Piovesan A, Pelleri MC, Antonaros F, Strippoli P, Caracausi M, Vitale L. On the length, weight and GC content of the human genome. *BMC Research Notes*. 2019;12(1). doi:https://doi.org/10.1186/s13104-019-4137-z

81. starr barry. A Long and Winding DNA. KQED. Published February 2, 2009. https://www.kqed.org/quest/1219/a-long-and-winding-dna

82. Ottman R. Gene–Environment Interaction: Definitions and Study Design. *Preventive Medicine*. 1996;25(6):764-770. doi:https://doi.org/10.1006/pmed.1996.0117

83. Ille AM, Lamont H, Mathews MB. The Central Dogma revisited: Insights from protein synthesis, CRISPR, and beyond. *WIREs RNA*. 2022;13(5). doi:https://doi.org/10.1002/wrna.1718

84. Haseltine WA, Patarca R. The RNA Revolution in the Central Molecular Biology Dogma Evolution. *International Journal of Molecular Sciences*. 2024;25(23):12695. doi:https://doi.org/10.3390/ijms252312695

85. Your Genome. How is DNA turned into protein? www.yourgenome.org. https://www.yourgenome.org/theme/how-is-dna-turned-into-protein-the-central-dogma-of-molecular-biology/

86. McManus M. Messenger RNA | McManus Lab. Ucsf.edu. Published 2021. https://mcmanuslab.ucsf.edu/node/276

87. Clancy S, Brown W. Translation: DNA to mRNA to Protein. Nature.com. Published 2008. https://www.nature.com/scitable/topicpage/translation-dna-to-mrna-to-protein-393/

88. LibreTexts. 4.1: Central Dogma of Molecular Biology. Biology LibreTexts. Published September 23, 2016. https://bio.libretexts.org/Bookshelves/Introductory_and_Ge neral_Biology/Introductory_Biology_(CK-12)/04:_Molecular_Biology/4.01:_Central_Dogma_of_Mol ecular_Biology

89. Wakim S, Grewal M. 6.4: Protein Synthesis. Biology LibreTexts. Published January 23, 2020. https://bio.libretexts.org/Bookshelves/Human_Biology/Hu man_Biology_(Wakim_and_Grewal)/06:_DNA_and_Prote in_Synthesis/6.04:_Protein_Synthesis

90. Hu L, Huang T, Liu XJ, Cai YD. Predicting Protein Phenotypes Based on Protein-Protein Interaction Network. Okazawa H, ed. *PLoS ONE*. 2011;6(3):e17668. doi:https://doi.org/10.1371/journal.pone.0017668

91. Toraño EG, García MG, Fernández-Morera JL, Niño-García P, Fernández AF. The Impact of External Factors on the Epigenome:In Uteroand over Lifetime. *BioMed Research International*. 2016;2016:1-17. doi:https://doi.org/10.1155/2016/2568635

92. CDC. Epigenetics, Health, and Disease. Genomics and Your Health. Published December 2, 2024.

https://www.cdc.gov/genomics-and-health/epigenetics/index.html

93. Breton CV, Landon R, Kahn LG, et al. Exploring the evidence for epigenetic regulation of environmental influences on child health across generations. *Communications Biology.* 2021;4(1). doi:https://doi.org/10.1038/s42003-021-02316-6

94. Coffin JM. 50th anniversary of the discovery of reverse transcriptase. Welch M, ed. *Molecular Biology of the Cell.* 2021;32(2):91-97. doi:https://doi.org/10.1091/mbc.e20-09-0612

95. Belfort M, Curcio MJ, Lue NF. Telomerase and retrotransposons: Reverse transcriptases that shaped genomes. *Proceedings of the National Academy of Sciences.* 2011;108(51):20304-20310. doi:https://doi.org/10.1073/pnas.1100269109

96. abcam. Reverse transcription: Process and applications | Abcam. Abcam.com. Published 2025. Accessed February 27, 2025. https://www.abcam.com/en-us/knowledge-center/dna-and-rna/rtpcr

97. Pray LA. The Biotechnology Revolution: PCR and Cloning Expressed Genes | Learn Science at Scitable. www.nature.com. Published 2008. https://www.nature.com/scitable/topicpage/the-biotechnology-revolution-pcr-and-the-use-553/

98. Menéndez-Arias L, Sebastián-Martín A, Álvarez M. Viral reverse transcriptases. *Virus Research.* 2017;234:153-176. doi:https://doi.org/10.1016/j.virusres.2016.12.019

99. ThermoFischer Scientific. Reverse Transcription Applications | Thermo Fisher Scientific - UK. Thermofisher.com. Published 2013. https://www.thermofisher.com/us/en/home/life-science/cloning/cloning-learning-center/invitrogen-school-of-molecular-biology/rt-education/reverse-transcription-applications.html

100. Baltimore D. Turning RNA Into DNA: The Discovery That Revolutionized Biology and Biotechnology. *Frontiers for Young Minds*. 2023;11. doi:https://doi.org/10.3389/frym.2023.1080663

101. Zittersteijn HA, Gonçalves MAFV, Hoeben RC. A primer to gene therapy: Progress, prospects, and problems. *Journal of Inherited Metabolic Disease*. 2021;44(1):54-71. doi:https://doi.org/10.1002/jimd.12270

102. NHS England. Non-coding DNA — Knowledge Hub. GeNotes. https://www.genomicseducation.hee.nhs.uk/genotes/knowledge-hub/non-coding-dna/

103. MedlinePlus. What is noncoding DNA?: MedlinePlus Genetics. medlineplus.gov. Published January 19, 2021. https://medlineplus.gov/genetics/understanding/basics/noncodingdna/

104. Levings D, Shaw KE, Lacher SE. Genomic Resources for Dissecting the Role of Non-Protein Coding Variation in Gene-Environment Interactions. *Toxicology*. 2020;441:152505. doi:https://doi.org/10.1016/j.tox.2020.152505

105. Lee T, Young Richard A. Transcriptional Regulation and Its Misregulation in Disease. *Cell.* 2013;152(6):1237-1251. doi:https://doi.org/10.1016/j.cell.2013.02.014

106. Doni Jayavelu N, Jajodia A, Mishra A, Hawkins RD. Candidate silencer elements for the human and mouse genomes. *Nature Communications.* 2020;11(1). doi:https://doi.org/10.1038/s41467-020-14853-5

107. Zhang Y, See YX, Tergaonkar V, Fullwood MJ. Long-Distance Repression by Human Silencers: Chromatin Interactions and Phase Separation in Silencers. *Cells.* 2022;11(9):1560. doi:https://doi.org/10.3390/cells11091560

108. Segert JA, Gisselbrecht SS, Bulyk ML. Transcriptional Silencers: Driving Gene Expression with the Brakes On. *Trends in Genetics.* 2021;37(6):514-527. doi:https://doi.org/10.1016/j.tig.2021.02.002

109. Newman T. Enzymes: Function, definition, and examples. www.medicalnewstoday.com. Published December 8, 2023. https://www.medicalnewstoday.com/articles/319704

110. Danaher. Exploring Restriction Enzymes | Restriction Endonuclease. Danaher Life Sciences. https://lifesciences.danaher.com/us/en/library/restriction-enzymes.html

111. Ni N. How Restriction Enzymes Changed Biology. The Scientist Magazine®. Published June 1, 2023. https://www.the-scientist.com/how-restriction-enzymes-changed-biology-71122

112. Wang X, Leptihn S. Defense and anti-defense mechanisms of bacteria and bacteriophages. *Journal of Zhejiang University Science B*. Published online February 14, 2024. doi:https://doi.org/10.1631/jzus.b2300101

113. Sigma Aldrich. NMR Chemical Shifts of Impurities. *Merck*. 2025;1(1). https://www.sigmaaldrich.com/MX/en/technical-documents/technical-article/genomics/cloning-and-expression/blue-white-screening

114. Gill J. How do phages block restriction enzymes? Tamu.edu. Published 2025. Accessed February 27, 2025. https://cpt.tamu.edu/491-research-projects/how-do-phages-block-restriction-enzymes/

115. LibreTexts. 6.3: Restriction Endonuclease. Chemistry LibreTexts. Published August 15, 2019. Accessed February 27, 2025. https://chem.libretexts.org/Courses/University_of_Arkansas_Little_Rock/CHEM_4320_5320:_Biochemistry_1/06:_Catalytic_Strategies_of_Enzymes/6.3:_Restriction_Endonuclease

116. Janscak P, MacWilliams MP, Sandmeier U, Nagaraja V, Bickle TA. DNA translocation blockage, a general mechanism of cleavage site selection by type I restriction enzymes. *The EMBO Journal*. 1999;18(9):2638-2647. doi:https://doi.org/10.1093/emboj/18.9.2638

117. Hazarika G, Dutta R, Saikia DP, et al. A comprehensive exploration of restriction enzymes and their applications in molecular biology: A review. *World Journal of Advanced*

Research and Reviews. 2024;21(1):2399-2404. doi:https://doi.org/10.30574/wjarr.2024.21.1.0269

118. Antonarakis SE, Phillips JA, Kazazian HH. Genetic diseases: diagnosis by restriction endonuclease analysis. *The Journal of Pediatrics.* 1982;100(6):845-856. doi:https://doi.org/10.1016/s0022-3476(82)80500-3

119. Sanford Health. Sanford PROMISE |Blog | Research Basics-Restriction Digest. Sanford Research. Published 2025. https://research.sanfordhealth.org/sanford-promise/blog/research-basics-restriction-digest

120. AAT Bioquest. What is the mechanism of DNA ligase? | AAT Bioquest. www.aatbio.com. Published March 26, 2024. https://www.aatbio.com/resources/faq-frequently-asked-questions/what-is-the-mechanism-of-dna-ligase

121. Danaher. DNA Ligation Overview: Mechanism, Types, Applications & Trends. Danaher Life Sciences. https://lifesciences.danaher.com/us/en/library/unveiling-dna-ligation.html

122. Doherty AJ. Structural and mechanistic conservation in DNA ligases. *Nucleic Acids Research.* 2000;28(21):4051-4058. doi:https://doi.org/10.1093/nar/28.21.4051

123. Sloan Kettering Institute. DNA Damage Recognition and Repair by DNA Ligases | Sloan Kettering Institute. www.mskcc.org. https://www.mskcc.org/research/ski/labs/stewart-shuman/dna-damage-recognition-and-repair-dna-ligases

124. Robb A, Zundel J. Point Mutations: Types, Processes & Effects | Study.com. Study.com. Published 2019.

https://study.com/academy/lesson/point-mutations-types-
processes-effects.html

125. Britannica. Point mutation | genetics | Britannica. In:
Encyclopædia Britannica. ; 2019.
https://www.britannica.com/science/point-mutation

126. Clancy S. Genetic Mutation. Scitable. Published 2008.
https://www.nature.com/scitable/topicpage/genetic-
mutation-441/

127. Petrosino M, Novak L, Pasquo A, et al. Analysis and
Interpretation of the Impact of Missense Variants in
Cancer. *International Journal of Molecular Sciences.*
2021;22(11):5416.
doi:https://doi.org/10.3390/ijms22115416

128. Hernández A. Missense Mutation: What Is It, Causes, and
More | Osmosis. www.osmosis.org. Published October 28,
2022. https://www.osmosis.org/answers/missense-mutation

129. Morais P, Adachi H, Yu YT. Suppression of Nonsense
Mutations by New Emerging Technologies. *International
Journal of Molecular Sciences.* 2020;21(12).
doi:https://doi.org/10.3390/ijms21124394

130. National Human Genome Research Institute. Nonsense
Mutation. Genome.gov. Published 2019.
https://www.genome.gov/genetics-glossary/Nonsense-
Mutation

131. Scitable. frameshift mutation / frame-shift mutation;
frameshift | Learn Science at Scitable. www.nature.com.
Published 2014.

https://www.nature.com/scitable/definition/frameshift-mutation-frame-shift-mutation-frameshift-203/

132.Cardiero G, Gennaro Musollino, Prezioso R, Lacerra G. mRNA Analysis of Frameshift Mutations with Stop Codon in the Last Exon: The Case of Hemoglobins Campania [α1 cod95 (–C)] and Sciacca [α1 cod109 (–C)]. *Biomedicines.* 2021;9(10):1390-1390. doi:https://doi.org/10.3390/biomedicines9101390

133.Sapkota A. Chromosomal Mutation- Definition, Causes, Mechanism, Types, Examples. Microbe Notes. Published March 11, 2021. https://microbenotes.com/chromosomal-mutation/

134.Pös O, Radvanszky J, Buglyó G, et al. DNA copy number variation: Main characteristics, evolutionary significance, and pathological aspects. *Biomedical Journal.* 2021;44(5):548-559. doi:https://doi.org/10.1016/j.bj.2021.02.003

135.Lobo I. Copy Number Variation and Genetic Disease | Learn Science at Scitable. www.nature.com. Published 2008. https://www.nature.com/scitable/topicpage/copy-number-variation-and-genetic-disease-911/

136.Zhou J, Lemos B, Dopman EB, Hartl DL. Copy-Number Variation: The Balance between Gene Dosage and Expression in Drosophila melanogaster. *Genome Biology and Evolution.* 2011;3:1014-1024. doi:https://doi.org/10.1093/gbe/evr023

137.Eichler E. Copy Number Variation and Human Disease | Learn Science at Scitable. www.nature.com.

https://www.nature.com/scitable/topicpage/copy-number-variation-and-human-disease-741737/

138. Tjandra K. Repeat Expansion Mutations More Common Than Thought | ALZFORUM. Alzforum.org. Published October 17, 2024. Accessed February 27, 2025. https://www.alzforum.org/news/research-news/repeat-expansion-mutations-more-common-thought

139. Paulson H. Repeat Expansion Diseases. *Neurogenetics, Part I.* 2018;147:105-123. doi:https://doi.org/10.1016/b978-0-444-63233-3.00009-9

140. Zhao W, Wang X, Li L, et al. Evaluation of environmental factors affecting the genetic diversity, genetic structure, and the potential distribution of Rhododendron aureum Georgi under changing climate. *Ecology and Evolution.* 2021;11(18):12294-12306. doi:https://doi.org/10.1002/ece3.7803

141. Rastogi RP, Richa, Kumar A, Tyagi MB, Sinha RP. Molecular Mechanisms of Ultraviolet Radiation-Induced DNA Damage and Repair. *Journal of Nucleic Acids.* 2010;2010(592980):1-32. doi:https://doi.org/10.4061/2010/592980

142. Rosendahl Huber A, Van Hoeck A, Van Boxtel R. The Mutagenic Impact of Environmental Exposures in Human Cells and Cancer: Imprints Through Time. *Frontiers in Genetics.* 2021;12. doi:https://doi.org/10.3389/fgene.2021.760039

143. Roychoudhury S, Jha NK, Ruokolainen J, Kesari KK. Mutagenic factors in the environment impacting human

and animal health. *Environmental Science and Pollution Research.* Published online August 2, 2022. doi:https://doi.org/10.1007/s11356-022-22247-x

144. Pulliero A, Cao J, Vasques L dos R, Pacchierotti F. Genetic and Epigenetic Effects of Environmental Mutagens and Carcinogens. *BioMed Research International.* 2015;2015. doi:https://doi.org/10.1155/2015/608054

145. Paoli J. HIV Resistant Mutation | Viruses101 | Learn Science at Scitable. Nature.com. Published 2013. https://www.nature.com/scitable/blog/viruses101/hiv_resist ant_mutation/

Chapter 4

146. Hunt K. How human gene editing is moving on after the CRISPR baby scandal. CNN. Published March 9, 2023. https://www.cnn.com/2023/03/09/health/genome-editing-crispr-whats-next-scn/index.html

147. Arturo Macarrón Palacios, Korus P, Bodo, Najmeh Heshmatpour, Patnaik SR. Revolutionizing in vivo therapy with CRISPR/Cas genome editing: breakthroughs, opportunities and challenges. *Frontiers in genome editing.* 2024;6. doi:https://doi.org/10.3389/fgeed.2024.1342193

148. Davis DJ, Sai. CRISPR Advancements for Human Health. *Missouri Medicine.* 2024;121(2):170. https://pmc.ncbi.nlm.nih.gov/articles/PMC11057861/

149. Asmamaw M, Zawdie B. Mechanism and Applications of CRISPR/Cas-9-Mediated Genome Editing. *Biologics :*

Targets & Therapy. 2021;15(1):353-361.
https://pmc.ncbi.nlm.nih.gov/articles/PMC8388126/

150.Chavez M, Chen X, Finn PB, Qi LS. Advances in CRISPR therapeutics. *Nature Reviews Nephrology.* 2022;19. doi:https://doi.org/10.1038/s41581-022-00636-2

151.Ran FA, Hsu PD, Wright J, Agarwala V, Scott DA, Zhang F. Genome engineering using the CRISPR-Cas9 system. *Nature Protocols.* 2013;8(11):2281-2308. https://www.nature.com/articles/nprot.2013.143

152.Balch B. Making science serve humanity: Jennifer Doudna, PhD, says CRISPR gene-editing technology should be accessible to all. AAMC. Published November 8, 2021. https://www.aamc.org/news/making-science-serve-humanity-jennifer-doudna-phd-says-crispr-gene-editing-technology-should-be

153.Henderson H. CRISPR clinical trials: a 2024 update. Innovative Genomics Institute (IGI). Published March 13, 2024. https://innovativegenomics.org/news/crispr-clinical-trials-2024/

154.Fernández CR. Seven diseases CRISPR technology could cure. Labiotech.eu. Published April 4, 2024. https://www.labiotech.eu/in-depth/crispr-technology-cure-disease/

155.Wold WSM, Toth K. Adenovirus vectors for gene therapy, vaccination and cancer gene therapy. *Current gene therapy.* 2013;13(6):421-433. doi:https://doi.org/10.2174/1566523213666131125095046

156.Kelsic ED, Church GM. Challenges and opportunities of machine-guided capsid engineering for gene therapy. *Cell and Gene Therapy Insights*. 2019;5(4):523-536. doi:https://doi.org/10.18609/cgti.2019.058

157.Bentler M, Hardet R, Ertelt M, et al. Modifying immune responses to adeno-associated virus vectors by capsid engineering. *Molecular Therapy - Methods & Clinical Development*. 2023;30:576-592. doi:https://doi.org/10.1016/j.omtm.2023.08.015

158.Wang D, Tai PWL, Gao G. Adeno-associated virus vector as a platform for gene therapy delivery. *Nature Reviews Drug Discovery*. 2019;18(5):358-378. doi:https://doi.org/10.1038/s41573-019-0012-9

159.Hastie E, Samulski RJ. Adeno-Associated Virus at 50: A Golden Anniversary of Discovery, Research, and Gene Therapy Success—A Personal Perspective. *Human Gene Therapy*. 2015;26(5):257-265. doi:https://doi.org/10.1089/hum.2015.025

160.Hysolli E. Gene Therapy: The Age of AAV. Wyss Institute. Published May 24, 2017. https://wyss.harvard.edu/news/gene-therapy-the-age-of-aav/

161.Au HKE, Isalan M, Mielcarek M. Gene Therapy Advances: A Meta-Analysis of AAV Usage in Clinical Settings. *Frontiers in Medicine*. 2022;8. doi:https://doi.org/10.3389/fmed.2021.809118

162.CBS News. Gene Therapy Helps Blind Boy See. Cbsnews.com. Published October 26, 2009. Accessed

March 5, 2025. https://www.cbsnews.com/news/gene-therapy-helps-blind-boy-see/

163. Simonelli F, Maguire AM, Testa F, et al. Gene Therapy for Leber's Congenital Amaurosis is Safe and Effective Through 1.5 Years After Vector Administration. *Molecular Therapy.* 2010;18(3):643-650. doi:https://doi.org/10.1038/mt.2009.277

164. Shea R. Curing Blindness, Part 1: Corey's Story. Foundation Fighting Blindness. Published 2025. Accessed March 5, 2025. https://www.fightingblindness.org/stories/curing-blindness-part-1-corey-s-story-44

165. Medline Plus. RPE65 gene: MedlinePlus Genetics. medlineplus.gov. https://medlineplus.gov/genetics/gene/rpe65/

166. Florian Udry, Decembrini S, Gamm DM, Déglon N, Kostic C, Yvan Arsenijévic. Lentiviral mediated RPE65 gene transfer in healthy hiPSCs-derived retinal pigment epithelial cells markedly increased RPE65 mRNA, but modestly protein level. *Scientific Reports.* 2020;10(1). doi:https://doi.org/10.1038/s41598-020-65657-y

167. Lewis R. Gene Therapy for Blindness Works! - DNA Science. DNA Science. Published May 7, 2015. Accessed March 5, 2025. https://dnascience.plos.org/2015/05/07/gene-therapy-for-blindness-works/

168. Drugs.com. Luxturna (voretigene neparvovec) FDA Approval History. Drugs.com. https://www.drugs.com/history/luxturna.html

169. Harvard.edu. Published 2017. Accessed March 5, 2025. https://eye.hms.harvard.edu/news/mass-eye-and-ear-performs-first-fda-approved-gene-therapy-procedure-inherited-disease

170. High K. AAV-mediated gene transfer for hemophilia. Published 2002. https://www.nature.com/articles/gim200289

171. Tarantino C. Coagulation Cascade: What Is It, Steps, and More | Osmosis. www.osmosis.org. Published November 8, 2021. https://www.osmosis.org/answers/coagulation-cascade

172. Perrin GQ, Herzog RW, Markusic DM. Update on clinical gene therapy for hemophilia. *Blood*. 2019;133(5):407-414. doi:https://doi.org/10.1182/blood-2018-07-820720

173. Batty P, Lillicrap D. Hemophilia Gene Therapy: Approaching the First Licensed Product. *HemaSphere*. 2021;5(3):e540. doi:https://doi.org/10.1097/hs9.0000000000000540

174. Fong S, Yates B, Sihn CR, et al. Interindividual variability in transgene mRNA and protein production following adeno-associated virus gene therapy for hemophilia A. *Nature Medicine*. 2022;28(4):789-797. doi:https://doi.org/10.1038/s41591-022-01751-0

175. Konkle BA, Walsh CE, Escobar MA, et al. BAX 335 hemophilia B gene therapy clinical trial results: potential impact of CpG sequences on gene expression. *Blood.* 2021;137(6):763-774. doi:https://doi.org/10.1182/blood.2019004625

176. Chowdary P, Shapiro S, Makris M, et al. Phase 1–2 Trial of AAVS3 Gene Therapy in Patients with Hemophilia B. *New England Journal of Medicine.* 2022;387(3):237-247. doi:https://doi.org/10.1056/nejmoa2119913

177. Nathwani AC, Reiss UM, Tuddenham EGD, et al. Long-term Safety and Efficacy of Factor IX Gene Therapy in Hemophilia B. *The New England journal of medicine.* 2014;371(21):1994-2004. doi:https://doi.org/10.1056/NEJMoa1407309

178. Christakopoulos GE, Telange R, Yen J, Weiss MJ. Gene Therapy and Gene Editing for β-Thalassemia. *Hematology/Oncology Clinics of North America.* 2023;37(2):433-447. doi:https://doi.org/10.1016/j.hoc.2022.12.012

179. Rosewell A, Vetrini F. Helper-Dependent Adenoviral Vectors. *Journal of Genetic Syndromes & Gene Therapy.* 2011;2(2). doi:https://doi.org/10.4172/2157-7412.s5-001

180. Lee D, Liu J, Junn HJ, Lee EJ, Jeong KS, Seol DW. No more helper adenovirus: production of gutless adenovirus (GLAd) free of adenovirus and replication-competent adenovirus (RCA) contaminants. *Experimental & Molecular Medicine.* 2019;51(10). doi:https://doi.org/10.1038/s12276-019-0334-z

181. Thacker EE, Timares L, Matthews QL. Strategies to overcome host immunity to adenovirus vectors in vaccine development. *Expert Review of Vaccines.* 2009;8(6):761-777. doi:https://doi.org/10.1586/erv.09.29

182. Aubert M, Strongin DE, Roychoudhury P, et al. Gene editing and elimination of latent herpes simplex virus in vivo. *Nature Communications.* 2020;11(1):4148. doi:https://doi.org/10.1038/s41467-020-17936-5

183. Epstein AL. HSV-1-derived amplicon vectors: recent technological improvements and remaining difficulties - a review. *Memórias do Instituto Oswaldo Cruz.* 2009;104(3):399-410. doi:https://doi.org/10.1590/s0074-02762009000300002

184. Jacobs A, Breakefield XO, Fraefel C. HSV-1-Based Vectors for Gene Therapy of Neurological Diseases and Brain Tumors: Part II. Vector Systems and Applications. *Neoplasia.* 1999;1(5):402-416. doi:https://doi.org/10.1038/sj.neo.7900056

185. Milone MC, O'Doherty U. Clinical Use of Lentiviral Vectors. *Leukemia.* 2018;32(7):1529-1541. doi:https://doi.org/10.1038/s41375-018-0106-0

186. Philadelphia TCH of. Emily Whitehead, First Pediatric Patient to Receive CAR T-Cell Therapy, Celebrates Cure 10 Years Later. www.chop.edu. Published May 10, 2022. https://www.chop.edu/news/emily-whitehead-first-pediatric-patient-receive-car-t-cell-therapy-celebrates-cure-10-years

187. Ghassemi S, Durgin JS, Nunez-Cruz S, et al. Rapid manufacturing of non-activated potent CAR T cells. *Nature Biomedical Engineering.* 2022;6(2):118-128. doi:https://doi.org/10.1038/s41551-021-00842-6

188. Lentiviral Vectors - the Application for CAR-T Therapies - Creative Biogene. Creative-biogene.com. Published 2017. https://www.creative-biogene.com/support/Lentiviral-Vectors-the-Application-for-CAR-T-Therapies

189. Ranzani M, Cesana D, Bartholomae CC, et al. Lentiviral vector–based insertional mutagenesis identifies genes associated with liver cancer. *Nature Methods.* 2013;10(2):155-161. doi:https://doi.org/10.1038/nmeth.2331

190. Schlimgen R, Howard J, Wooley D, et al. Risks Associated With Lentiviral Vector Exposures and Prevention Strategies. *Journal of Occupational and Environmental Medicine.* 2016;58(12):1159-1166. doi:https://doi.org/10.1097/JOM.0000000000000879

191. Modlich U, Baum C. Preventing and exploiting the oncogenic potential of integrating gene vectors. *Journal of Clinical Investigation.* 2009;119(4):755-758. doi:https://doi.org/10.1172/jci38831

192. Bona R, Michelini Z, Mazzei C, et al. Safety and efficiency modifications of SIV-based integrase-defective lentiviral vectors for immunization. *Molecular Therapy Methods & Clinical Development.* 2021;23:263. doi:https://doi.org/10.1016/j.omtm.2021.09.011

193. Lundstrom K. Alphaviruses in Cancer Therapy. *Frontiers in Molecular Biosciences*. 2022;9. doi:https://doi.org/10.3389/fmolb.2022.864781

194. UHBlog. Clinical Trial Studies Treating Brain Tumor with Genetically Modified Poliovirus. Uhhospitals.org. Published January 27, 2020. Accessed March 5, 2025. https://www.uhhospitals.org/blog/articles/2020/01/clinical-trial-studies-treating-brain-tumor-with-genetically-modified-poliovirus

195. Duke University. Duke Study: Poliovirus Therapy for Recurrent Glioblastoma Has 3-Year Survival Rate of 21%. Duke Department of Neurosurgery. Published June 26, 2018. Accessed March 5, 2025. https://neurosurgery.duke.edu/news/duke-study-poliovirus-therapy-recurrent-glioblastoma-has-3-year-survival-rate-21

196. Fox M, Dunn L. A new use for polio vaccine: Fighting brain tumors. NBC News. Published June 27, 2018. https://www.nbcnews.com/health/health-news/modified-polio-vaccine-helps-fight-deadly-brain-tumors-n886486

197. Duke University. Update on Recombinant Poliovirus Cancer Immunotherapy | Tisch Brain Tumor Center. tischbraintumorcenter.duke.edu. https://tischbraintumorcenter.duke.edu/stories/update-recombinant-poliovirus-cancer-immunotherapy

198. Duke University. First patient to undergo poliovirus therapy for GBM dies eight years after treatment. Duke Department of Neurosurgery. Published April 6, 2020. Accessed March 5, 2025.

https://neurosurgery.duke.edu/news/first-patient-undergo-poliovirus-therapy-gbm-dies-eight-years-after-treatment

199. Zhao Y, Huang L. Lipid Nanoparticles for Gene Delivery. *Nonviral Vectors for Gene Therapy - Lipid- and Polymer-based Gene Transfer.* 2014;88:13-36. doi:https://doi.org/10.1016/b978-0-12-800148-6.00002-x

200. Duan L, Ouyang K, Xu X, et al. Nanoparticle Delivery of CRISPR/Cas9 for Genome Editing. *Frontiers in Genetics.* 2021;12. doi:https://doi.org/10.3389/fgene.2021.673286

201. Chen L. Lipid Nanoparticles: A Breakthrough in CRISPR Delivery Systems | GenScript. Genscript.com. Published 2024. https://www.genscript.com/lipid-nanoparticles-the-vanguard-of-crispr-delivery-systems.html

202. Hou X, Zaks T, Langer R, Dong Y. Lipid nanoparticles for mRNA delivery. *Nature Reviews Materials.* 2021;6(6):1078-1094. doi:https://doi.org/10.1038/s41578-021-00358-0

203. ThermoFisher. mRNA Delivery Technology | Thermo Fisher Scientific - US. Thermofisher.com. Published 2024. https://www.thermofisher.com/us/en/home/references/gibco-cell-culture-basics/transfection-basics/applications/mrna-delivery.html

204. ThermoFisher. Duration of siRNA Induced Silencing: Your Questions Answered | Thermo Fisher Scientific - US. Thermofisher.com. Published 2024. https://www.thermofisher.com/us/en/home/references/amb

ion-tech-support/rnai-sirna/tech-notes/duration-of-sirna-induced-silencing.html

205. Cross R. Without these lipid shells, there would be no mRNA vaccines for COVID-19. Acs.org. Published March 6, 2021. https://cen.acs.org/pharmaceuticals/drug-delivery/Without-lipid-shells-mRNA-vaccines/99/i8

206. Swetha K, Kotla NG, Tunki L, et al. Recent Advances in the Lipid Nanoparticle-Mediated Delivery of mRNA Vaccines. *Vaccines*. 2023;11(3):658. doi:https://doi.org/10.3390/vaccines11030658

207. Merck KGaA. Lipids: Protecting mRNA so it can protect our body. Emdgroup.com. Published 2020. https://www.emdgroup.com/en/research/science-space/envisioning-tomorrow/precision-medicine/lipid-nanoparticles.html

208. Agrawal N, Dasaradhi PVN, Mohmmed A, Malhotra P, Bhatnagar RK, Mukherjee SK. RNA Interference: Biology, Mechanism, and Applications. *Microbiology and Molecular Biology Reviews*. 2003;67(4):657-685. doi:https://doi.org/10.1128/mmbr.67.4.657-685.2003

209. NCBI. RNA Interference (RNAi). Nih.gov. Published 2017. https://www.ncbi.nlm.nih.gov/probe/docs/techrnai/

210. ThermoFisher. Gene Specific Silencing by RNAi - US. www.thermofisher.com. https://www.thermofisher.com/us/en/home/references/ambion-tech-support/rnai-sirna/tech-notes/gene-specific-silencing-by-rnai.html

211. Khorkova O, Stahl J, Joji A, Volmar CH, Wahlestedt C. Amplifying gene expression with RNA-targeted therapeutics. *Nature Reviews Drug Discovery*. 2023;22(7):539-561. doi:https://doi.org/10.1038/s41573-023-00704-7

212. Hawkins PG, Morris KV. RNA and transcriptional modulation of gene expression. *Cell Cycle*. 2008;7(5):602-607. doi:https://doi.org/10.4161/cc.7.5.5522

213. Mount Sinai. Gene Splicing for Therapeutic Use. reports.mountsinai.org. https://reports.mountsinai.org/article/tisch2021-10-guccione

214. Zhu Y, Zhu L, Wang X, Jin H. RNA-based therapeutics: an overview and prospectus. *Cell Death & Disease*. 2022;13(7):1-15. doi:https://doi.org/10.1038/s41419-022-05075-2

215. Regenerative in. IVT mRNA in Regenerative Medicine. Biocompare.com. Published August 8, 2023. Accessed March 6, 2025. https://www.biocompare.com/Editorial-Articles/598366-IVT-mRNA-in-Regenerative-Medicine/

216. Xu Y, Qiu M, Shen M, et al. The emerging regulatory roles of long non-coding RNAs implicated in cancer metabolism. *Molecular Therapy*. 2021;29(7):2209-2218. doi:https://doi.org/10.1016/j.ymthe.2021.03.017

217. Qian Y, Shi L, Luo Z. Long Non-coding RNAs in Cancer: Implications for Diagnosis, Prognosis, and Therapy. *Frontiers in Medicine*. 2020;7. doi:https://doi.org/10.3389/fmed.2020.612393

218. Julia-Sophia Bellingrath, McClements ME, Fischer M, MacLaren RE. Programmable RNA editing with endogenous ADAR enzymes – a feasible option for the treatment of inherited retinal disease? *Frontiers in Molecular Neuroscience*. 2023;16. doi:https://doi.org/10.3389/fnmol.2023.1092913

219. Savva YA, Rieder LE, Reenan RA. The ADAR protein family. *Genome Biology*. 2012;13(12):252. doi:https://doi.org/10.1186/gb-2012-13-12-252

220. Booth BJ, Sami Nourreddine, Dhruva Katrekar, et al. RNA editing: Expanding the potential of RNA therapeutics. *Molecular Therapy*. 2023;31(6). doi:https://doi.org/10.1016/j.ymthe.2023.01.005

221. Anderson S. Gene editing: DNA versus RNA. Drug Discover NewsDrug Discovery News, Development & Diagnostics Articles | DDN Magazine. Published February 14, 2023. Accessed March 6, 2025. https://www.drugdiscoverynews.com/gene-editing-dna-versus-rna-15618

222. Hui F, Liu GSR. RNA editing is the next frontier in gene therapy – here's what you need to know. The Conversation. Published November 21, 2024. https://theconversation.com/rna-editing-is-the-next-frontier-in-gene-therapy-heres-what-you-need-to-know-243938

223. Shah-Neville W. RNA editing set to take off: could DNA's short-lived cousin overcome the limitations of CRISPR gene editing? Labiotech.eu. Published February 12, 2024.

https://www.labiotech.eu/in-depth/rna-editing-reaches-clinic/

224. Telangana Today. Genome editing, a game-changer for treating genetic disorders: Expert. Telangana Today. Published June 27, 2023. Accessed March 6, 2025. https://telanganatoday.com/genome-editing-a-game-changer-for-treating-genetic-disorders-expert

225. Chou ST ., Leng Q, Mixson J. Zinc finger nucleases: Tailor-made for gene therapy. *Drugs of the Future*. 2012;37(3):183. doi:https://doi.org/10.1358/dof.2012.037.03.1779022

226. Rahman SH, Maeder ML, Joung JK, Cathomen T. Zinc-Finger Nucleases for Somatic Gene Therapy: The Next Frontier. *Human Gene Therapy*. 2011;22(8):925-933. doi:https://doi.org/10.1089/hum.2011.087

227. Li H, Yang Y, Hong W, Huang M, Wu M, Zhao X. Applications of genome editing technology in the targeted therapy of human diseases: mechanisms, advances and prospects. *Signal Transduction and Targeted Therapy*. 2020;5(1):1-23. doi:https://doi.org/10.1038/s41392-019-0089-y

228. Carroll D. Genome Engineering With Zinc-Finger Nucleases. *Genetics*. 2011;188(4):773-782. doi:https://doi.org/10.1534/genetics.111.131433

229. Carroll D. Progress and prospects: Zinc-finger nucleases as gene therapy agents. *Gene Therapy*. 2008;15(22):1463-1468. doi:https://doi.org/10.1038/gt.2008.145

230. Swarthout JT, Raisinghani M, Cui X. Zinc Finger Nucleases: A new era for transgenic animals. *Annals Of Neurosciences.* 2011;18(1). doi:https://doi.org/10.5214/ans.0972.7531.1118109

231. Yeadon J. Pros and cons of ZNFs, TALENs, and CRISPR/Cas. The Jackson Laboratory. Published March 4, 2014. https://www.jax.org/news-and-insights/jax-blog/2014/march/pros-and-cons-of-znfs-talens-and-crispr-cas

232. clinicalinfo.hiv.gov. SB-728-T Health Professional Drug Record | NIH. Hiv.gov. Published 2021. https://clinicalinfo.hiv.gov/en/drugs/sb-728-t/health-professional

233. Ashmore-Harris C, Fruhwirth GO. The clinical potential of gene editing as a tool to engineer cell-based therapeutics. *Clinical and Translational Medicine.* 2020;9(1). doi:https://doi.org/10.1186/s40169-020-0268-z

234. Anguela XM, Sharma R, Doyon Y, et al. Robust ZFN-mediated genome editing in adult hemophilic mice. *Blood.* 2013;122(19):3283-3287. doi:https://doi.org/10.1182/blood-2013-04-497354

235. NHS England. Phase 1 Gene Therapy study of SB-FIX in Severe Haemophilia B. Health Research Authority. Published 2020. Accessed March 6, 2025. https://www.hra.nhs.uk/planning-and-improving-research/application-summaries/research-summaries/phase-1-gene-therapy-study-of-sb-fix-in-severe-haemophilia-b/

236. Sangamo Therapeutics, Inc. New strategies for optimizing the specificity of gene editing nucleases. Phys.org. Published July 30, 2019. Accessed March 6, 2025. https://phys.org/news/2019-07-strategies-optimizing-specificity-gene-nucleases.html

237. Paschon DE, Lussier S, Wangzor T, et al. Diversifying the structure of zinc finger nucleases for high-precision genome editing. *Nature Communications.* 2019;10(1). doi:https://doi.org/10.1038/s41467-019-08867-x

238. Joung JK, Sander JD. TALENs: a widely applicable technology for targeted genome editing. *Nature Reviews Molecular Cell Biology.* 2012;14(1):49-55. doi:https://doi.org/10.1038/nrm3486

239. ThermoFisher. TALEN Technology Information - US. www.thermofisher.com. https://www.thermofisher.com/us/en/home/life-science/genome-editing/genome-editing-learning-center/designer-talen-technology-information.html

240. Boch J. TALEN Technology Information - US. www.thermofisher.com. https://www.thermofisher.com/us/en/home/life-science/genome-editing/genome-editing-learning-center/designer-talen-technology-information.html

241. Xia E, Zhang Y, Cao H, Li J, Duan R, Hu J. Genes | Free Full-Text | TALEN-Mediated Gene Targeting for Cystic Fibrosis-Gene Therapy. Mdpi.com. Published 2019. Accessed March 6, 2025. https://www.mdpi.com/2073-4425/10/1/39/review_report

242. Xia E, Zhang Y, Cao H, Li J, Duan R, Hu J. TALEN-Mediated Gene Targeting for Cystic Fibrosis-Gene Therapy. *Genes.* 2019;10(1):39. doi:https://doi.org/10.3390/genes10010039

243. ThermoFisher. TALEN Gene Editing - US. www.thermofisher.com. https://www.thermofisher.com/us/en/home/life-science/genome-editing/talens.html

244. ISAAA. COVID-19 Treatment Efforts Using Plant Technologies. ISAAA. https://www.isaaa.org/resources/publications/pocketk/59/default.asp

Chapter 5

245. Rady Children's Institute for Genomic Medicine. Fitz's Story | RCIGM. RCIGM. Published October 10, 2024. https://radygenomics.org/case-studies/fitzs-story/

246. Fischer A, Hacein-Bey-Abina S. Gene therapy for severe combined immunodeficiencies and beyond. *The Journal of Experimental Medicine.* 2019;217(2). doi:https://doi.org/10.1084/jem.20190607

247. Pavel-Dinu M, Wiebking V, Dejene BT, et al. Gene correction for SCID-X1 in long-term hematopoietic stem cells. *Nature Communications.* 2019;10(1). doi:https://doi.org/10.1038/s41467-019-09614-y

248. UCSF Benioff Children's Hospitals. UCSF Benioff Children's Hospital. www.ucsfbenioffchildrens.org. https://www.ucsfbenioffchildrens.org/

249. Powers MP. Newborn Screening: 60 Years and Counting. APHL. https://www.aphl.org/aboutAPHL/publications/lab-matters/Pages/Newborn-Screening-60-Years-and-Counting.aspx

250. Rady Children's Institute for Genomic Medicine. Sequence of Hope: Fitz's Story | Rady Children's Hospital Foundation. Rady Children's Hospital Foundation |. Published May 16, 2023. https://radyfoundation.org/blog/fitzs-story/

251. Wu C, Lu H, Cassis LA, Daugherty A. Molecular and Pathophysiological Features of Angiotensinogen: A Mini Review. *American Chinese Journal of Medicine and Science*. 2011;4(4):183. doi:https://doi.org/10.7156/v4i4p183

252. Förstermann U, Sessa WC. Nitric oxide synthases: regulation and function. *European heart journal*. 2012;33(7):829-837, 837a837d. doi:https://doi.org/10.1093/eurheartj/ehr304

253. Evangelou E, Warren HR, Mosen-Ansorena D, et al. Genetic analysis of over 1 million people identifies 535 new loci associated with blood pressure traits. *Nature Genetics*. 2018;50(10):1412-1425. doi:https://doi.org/10.1038/s41588-018-0205-x

254. Bousseau S, Fais RS, Gu S, Frump A, Lahm T. Pathophysiology and new advances in pulmonary hypertension. *BMJ Medicine*. 2023;2(1). doi:https://doi.org/10.1136/bmjmed-2022-000137

255. Ma J, Chen X. Advances in pathogenesis and treatment of essential hypertension. *Frontiers in Cardiovascular Medicine.* 2022;9. doi:https://doi.org/10.3389/fcvm.2022.1003852

256. Vrablik M, Dlouha D, Todorovova V, Stefler D, Hubacek JA. Genetics of Cardiovascular Disease: How Far Are We from Personalized CVD Risk Prediction and Management? *International Journal of Molecular Sciences.* 2021;22(8):4182. doi:https://doi.org/10.3390/ijms22084182

257. Bao M, Li P, Li Q, et al. Genetic screening for monogenic hypertension in hypertensive individuals in a clinical setting. *Journal of Medical Genetics.* 2020;57(8):571-580. doi:https://doi.org/10.1136/jmedgenet-2019-106145

258. Qi Q, Forman JP, Jensen MK, et al. Genetic Predisposition to High Blood Pressure Associates With Cardiovascular Complications Among Patients With Type 2 Diabetes: Two Independent Studies. *Diabetes.* 2012;61(11):3026-3032. doi:https://doi.org/10.2337/db12-0225

259. Medline Plus. CYP2C19 gene: MedlinePlus Genetics. medlineplus.gov. https://medlineplus.gov/genetics/gene/cyp2c19/

260. Flaten HK, Kim HS, Campbell J, Hamilton L, Monte AA. CYP2C19 drug-drug and drug-gene interactions in ED patients,,. *The American journal of emergency medicine.* 2016;34(2):245-249. doi:https://doi.org/10.1016/j.ajem.2015.10.055

261. Children's Minnesota. Cytochrome P450 2C19 (CYP2C19) Rapid Metabolizer. Children's Minnesota. https://www.childrensmn.org/educationmaterials/childrens mn/article/17875/cytochrome-p450-2c19-cyp2c19-rapid-metabolizer/

262. Mahmood Mahajna, Rami Abu Fanne, Matitiahu Berkovitch, et al. Effect of CYP2C19 Pharmacogenetic Testing on Predicting Citalopram and Escitalopram Tolerability and Efficacy: A Retrospective, Longitudinal Cohort Study. *Biomedicines.* 2023;11(12):3245-3245. doi:https://doi.org/10.3390/biomedicines11123245

263. Nilupaer Shafeng, Han D, Ma Y, Abudusalamu R, Binuer Ayitimuhan. Association between the HLA-B*1502 gene and mild maculopapular exanthema induced by antiepileptic drugs in Northwest China. *BMC neurology.* 2021;21(1). doi:https://doi.org/10.1186/s12883-021-02363-w

264. Ferrell PB, McLeod HL. Carbamazepine, HLA-B*1502 and risk of Stevens-Johnson syndrome and toxic epidermal necrolysis: US FDA recommendations. *Pharmacogenomics.* 2008;9(10):1543-1546. doi:https://doi.org/10.2217/14622416.9.10.1543

265. Boxcar Studio. Genetic Testing is Key to Safer Chemotherapy | UM College of Pharmacy. Umich.edu. Published 2022. https://pharmacy.umich.edu/about-college/news/category/blog/genetic-testing-key-safer-chemotherapy

266. Moen EL, Godley LA, Zhang W, Dolan ME. Pharmacogenomics of chemotherapeutic susceptibility

and toxicity. *Genome Medicine.* 2012;4(11):90.
doi:https://doi.org/10.1186/gm391

267. California AZ PharmD Clinical Pharmacist Cedars Sinai
Medical Network Beverly Hills, California John Andraos,
PharmD Clinical Pharmacist Cedars Sinai Medical
Network Beverly Hills, California Ajay Sharma, BPharm,
PhD Assistant Professor of Pharmacology Chapman
University School of Pharmacy Irvine, California Moom
R. Roosan, PharmD, PhD Assistant Professor Chapman
University School of Pharmacy Irvine. Pharmacogenomic
Considerations in Opioid Therapy.
www.uspharmacist.com.
https://www.uspharmacist.com/article/pharmacogenomic-
considerations-in-opioid-therapy

268. Cleveland Clinic. Cochlear Implants. Cleveland Clinic.
Published March 23, 2023.
https://my.clevelandclinic.org/health/treatments/4806-
cochlear-implants

269. Pangršič T, Reisinger E, Moser T. Otoferlin: a multi-C2
domain protein essential for hearing. *Trends in
Neurosciences.* 2012;35(11):671-680.
doi:https://doi.org/10.1016/j.tins.2012.08.002

270. Regeneron Pharmaceuticals. Latest DB-OTO Results
Show Dramatically Improved Hearing to Normal Levels
in a Child with Profound Genetic Deafness within 24
Weeks and Initial Hearing Improvements in a Second
Child at 6 Weeks | Regeneron Pharmaceuticals Inc.
Regeneron Pharmaceuticals Inc. Published 2024.
https://investor.regeneron.com/news-releases/news-release-

details/latest-db-oto-results-show-dramatically-improved-hearing-normal

271. NHS England. Baby born deaf can hear after breakthrough gene therapy. Cambridge University Hospitals. https://www.cuh.nhs.uk/news/baby-born-deaf-can-hear-after-breakthrough-gene-therapy/

272. Hacein-Bey-Abina S, Garrigue A, Wang GP, et al. Insertional oncogenesis in 4 patients after retrovirus-mediated gene therapy of SCID-X1. *Journal of Clinical Investigation*. 2008;118(9):3132-3142. doi:https://doi.org/10.1172/jci35700

273. Check E. A tragic setback. *Nature*. 2002;420(6912):116-118. doi:https://doi.org/10.1038/420116a

274. Ruggero K, Al-Assar O, Chambers JS, Codrington R, Brend T, Rabbitts TH. LMO2 and IL2RG synergize in thymocytes to mimic the evolution of SCID-X1 gene therapy-associated T-cell leukaemia. *Leukemia*. 2016;30(9):1959-1962. doi:https://doi.org/10.1038/leu.2016.116

275. McCormack MP, A. Förster, Drynan L, Pannell R, Rabbitts TH. The *LMO2* T-Cell Oncogene Is Activated via Chromosomal Translocations or Retroviral Insertion during Gene Therapy but Has No Mandatory Role in Normal T-Cell Development. *Molecular and Cellular Biology*. 2003;23(24):9003-9013. doi:https://doi.org/10.1128/mcb.23.24.9003-9013.2003

276. Davé UP, Akagi K, Tripathi R, et al. Murine Leukemias with Retroviral Insertions at Lmo2 Are Predictive of the

Leukemias Induced in SCID-X1 Patients Following Retroviral Gene Therapy. Horwitz MS, ed. *PLoS Genetics*. 2009;5(5):e1000491. doi:https://doi.org/10.1371/journal.pgen.1000491

277. Williams DA, Thrasher AJ. Concise Review: Lessons Learned From Clinical Trials of Gene Therapy in Monogenic Immunodeficiency Diseases. *STEM CELLS Translational Medicine*. 2014;3(5):636-642. doi:https://doi.org/10.5966/sctm.2013-0206

278. Cavazzana M, Six E, Lagresle-Peyrou C, André-Schmutz I, Hacein-Bey-Abina S. Gene Therapy for X-Linked Severe Combined Immunodeficiency: Where Do We Stand? *Human gene therapy*. 2016;27(2):108-116. doi:https://doi.org/10.1089/hum.2015.137

279. Kohn DB, Chen YY, Spencer MJ. Successes and Challenges in Clinical Gene Therapy. *Gene Therapy*. 2023;30:1-9. doi:https://doi.org/10.1038/s41434-023-00390-5

280. CANAVAN FOUNDATION. About Canavan Disease | Canavan Foundation. www.canavanfoundation.org. https://www.canavanfoundation.org/about_canavan_disease

281. CANaspire - A Clinical Trial for Canavan Disease. Developing a Canavan Treatment | Aspa Clinical Trials. Published March 2023. https://treatcanavan.com/canaspire-trial/

282. Medline Plus. ASPA gene: MedlinePlus Genetics. medlineplus.gov. https://medlineplus.gov/genetics/gene/aspa/

283. Spencer SEW. Family connects with researchers behind Canavan gene therapy. UMass Chan Medical School. Published July 18, 2023. https://www.umassmed.edu/news/news-archives/2023/07/family-connects-with-researchers-behind-canavan-gene-therapy/

284. National Heart, Lung, and Blood Institute. Sickle Cell Disease - What is Sickle Cell Disease? www.nhlbi.nih.gov. Published September 30, 2024. https://www.nhlbi.nih.gov/health/sickle-cell-disease

285. CHOP. Children's Hospital of Philadelphia. Chop.edu. Published 2019. https://www.chop.edu/

286. Philadelphia TCH of. Gene Therapy for Sickle Cell Disease: Marie-Chantal's Story. www.chop.edu. Published November 22, 2023. https://www.chop.edu/stories/gene-therapy-sickle-cell-disease-marie-chantal-s-story

287. National Human Genome Research Institute. About Sickle Cell Disease. National Human Genome Research Institute. Published May 26, 2020. https://www.genome.gov/Genetic-Disorders/Sickle-Cell-Disease

288. Nagalla S, Ballas SK. Drugs for preventing red blood cell dehydration in people with sickle cell disease. *Cochrane Database of Systematic Reviews*. Published online

October 19, 2018.
doi:https://doi.org/10.1002/14651858.cd003426.pub6

289.Vertex Pharmaceuticals Incorporated. Vertex and CRISPR Therapeutics Announce US FDA Approval of CASGEVY™.… CRISPR Therapeutics. https://crisprtx.com/about-us/press-releases-and-presentations/vertex-and-crispr-therapeutics-announce-us-fda-approval-of-casgevy-exagamglogene-autotemcel-for-the-treatment-of-sickle-cell-disease

290.Kwilas A. *Summary Basis for Regulatory Action.*; 2023. Accessed February 24, 2025. https://www.fda.gov/media/175179/download

Chapter 6

291.Zoulikha Rezoug, Totten SP, Szlachtycz D, et al. Universal Genetic Testing for Newly Diagnosed Invasive Breast Cancer. *JAMA Network Open.* 2024;7(9):e2431427-e2431427. doi:https://doi.org/10.1001/jamanetworkopen.2024.31427

292.CDC. Real Stories About Lynch Syndrome. Hereditary Colorectal (Colon) Cancer. Published October 16, 2024. https://www.cdc.gov/colorectal-cancer-hereditary/stories/index.html

293.Medline Plus. What are the benefits of genetic testing? medlineplus.gov. Published September 17, 2020. https://medlineplus.gov/genetics/understanding/testing/benefits/

294.Varghese SE, Otol RHME, Olama FSA, Elbadawi SAM. The Importance of Early Detection of Genetic Diseases.

Dubai Medical Journal. 2021;4(2):133-141. doi:https://doi.org/10.1159/000514215

295. Travis J. How a geneticist led the effort to free a mother convicted of killing her kids. www.science.org. Published June 3, 2023. https://www.science.org/content/article/how-geneticist-led-effort-free-mother-convicted-killing-her-kids

296. Housden T. Kathleen Folbigg: Woman jailed over infant deaths pardoned. *BBC News.* https://www.bbc.com/news/world-australia-65806606. Published June 5, 2023.

297. Aguera J. Genetics, truth and justice. reporter.anu.edu.au. Published December 14, 2023. https://reporter.anu.edu.au/all-stories/genetics-truth-and-justice

298. Baker H. Australia's "worst female serial killer" freed after her children's deadly gene mutations come to light. livescience.com. Published June 15, 2023. Accessed February 25, 2025. https://www.livescience.com/health/genetics/australias-worst-female-serial-killer-freed-after-her-childrens-deadly-gene-mutations-come-to-light

299. Collins FS, Green ED, Guttmacher AE, Guyer MS. A vision for the future of genomics research. *Nature.* 2003;422(6934):835-847. doi:https://doi.org/10.1038/nature01626

300. Hazel JW, Clayton EW. Law Enforcement and Genetic Data. The Hastings Center. Published January 20, 2021.

https://www.thehastingscenter.org/briefingbook/law-enforcement-and-genetic-data/

301.Bryan K. Lawmakers Cautious as Genetic Tests Help in Cracking Cold Cases. National Conference of State Legislatures. Published October 23, 2023. https://www.ncsl.org/state-legislatures-news/details/lawmakers-cautious-as-genetic-tests-help-in-cracking-cold-cases

302.Blender D. *American Abyss: Savagery and Civilization in the Age of Industry.* Cornell University Press; 2011.

303.National Human Genome Research Institute. Eugenics and Scientific Racism. National Human Genome Research Institute. Published May 18, 2022. https://www.genome.gov/about-genomics/fact-sheets/Eugenics-and-Scientific-Racism

304.Stern AM. Eugenics, sterilization, and historical memory in the United States. *História, Ciências, Saúde-Manguinhos.* 2016;23(suppl 1):195-212. doi:https://doi.org/10.1590/s0104-59702016000500011

305.Jackson CS, Turner D, June M, Miller MV. Facing Our History—Building an Equitable Future. *The American Journal of Human Genetics.* 2023;110(3):377-395. doi:https://doi.org/10.1016/j.ajhg.2023.02.005

306.Cohen A. The Supreme Court Ruling That Led To 70,000 Forced Sterilizations. NPR.org. Published March 7, 2016. https://www.npr.org/sections/health-shots/2016/03/07/469478098/the-supreme-court-ruling-that-led-to-70-000-forced-sterilizations

307.Garver KL, Garver B. Eugenics: past, present, and the future. *American Journal of Human Genetics.* 1991;49(5):1109. https://pmc.ncbi.nlm.nih.gov/articles/PMC1683254/

308.Oklahoma Eugenics. Uvm.edu. Published 2010. https://www.uvm.edu/~lkaelber/eugenics/OK/OK.html

309.Ko L. Unwanted Sterilization and Eugenics Programs in the United States. Independent Lens. Published January 29, 2016. https://www.pbs.org/independentlens/blog/unwanted-sterilization-and-eugenics-programs-in-the-united-states/

310.Berenbaum M. T4 Program | Definition and History. In: *Encyclopædia Britannica.* ; 2018. https://www.britannica.com/event/T4-Program

311.United States Holocaust Memorial Museum. Euthanasia Program and Aktion T4. Ushmm.org. Published October 7, 2020. https://encyclopedia.ushmm.org/content/en/article/euthanasia-program

312.Holocaust Memorial Day Trust. Holocaust Memorial Day Trust | Disabled people. Hmd.org.uk. Published 2024. https://hmd.org.uk/learn-about-the-holocaust-and-genocides/nazi-persecution/disabled-people/

313.Nowak K. Annual 4 Chapter 14. www.museumoftolerance.com. https://www.museumoftolerance.com/education/archives-and-reference-library/online-resources/simon-wiesenthal-center-annual-volume-4/annual-4-chapter-14.html

314. Lenartz A, Scherer AM, Uhlmann WR, Suter SM, Anderson Hartley C, Prince AER. The persistent lack of knowledge and misunderstanding of the Genetic Information Nondiscrimination Act (GINA) more than a decade after passage. *Genetics in Medicine: Official Journal of the American College of Medical Genetics*. 2021;23(12):2324-2334. doi:https://doi.org/10.1038/s41436-021-01268-w

315. Medosch E. Not Just ICE: Forced Sterilization in the United States | Immigration and Human Rights Law Review. Immigration and Human Rights Law Review. Published May 28, 2021. https://lawblogs.uc.edu/ihrlr/2021/05/28/not-just-ice-forced-sterilization-in-the-united-states/

316. National Human Genome Research Institute (NHGRI). Genetic Information Nondiscrimination Act (GINA). Genome.gov. https://www.genome.gov/genetics-glossary/Genetic-Information-Nondiscrimination-Act

317. National Human Genome Research Institute. Genetic Discrimination. Genome.gov. Published January 6, 2022. https://www.genome.gov/about-genomics/policy-issues/Genetic-Discrimination

318. The Coppola Firm. HR Alert: ADA and GINA Compliance in the Hiring Process - The Coppola Firm. The Coppola Firm - Attorneys & Counselors At Law. Published November 6, 2023. Accessed February 25, 2025. https://coppolalegal.com/2023/11/hr-alert-ada-and-gina-compliance-in-the-hiring-process/

319. Thomas S. Dollar General to pay $1 million for genetic information and disability discrimination. www.hcamag.com. Published October 23, 2023. https://www.hcamag.com/us/specialization/diversity-inclusion/dollar-general-to-pay-1-million-for-genetic-information-and-disability-discrimination/464384

320. CBS. Jury awards millions in case of the "devious defecator." Cbsnews.com. Published June 25, 2015. Accessed February 25, 2025. https://www.cbsnews.com/news/jury-awards-millions-in-case-of-the-devious-defecator/

321. The National Trial Lawyers. Employees Recover $2.2M in "Devious Defecator" DNA Swab Case. National Trial Lawyers. Published 2023. https://thenationaltriallawyers.org/article/devious-defecator/

322. Brown K. 23andMe Hack Breaches 6.9 Million Users' Info, Including Some's Health Data. TIME. Published December 4, 2023. https://time.com/6342551/23andme-hack-health-data-profiles-compromised/

323. 23andMe. Addressing Data Security Concerns. 23andMe Blog. Published October 7, 2023. https://blog.23andme.com/articles/addressing-data-security-concerns

324. Joyce. 23andMe Data Breach - California Lawyers Association. California Lawyers Association. Published January 25, 2024. https://calawyers.org/privacy-law/23andme-data-breach/

325. Franceschi-Bicchierai L. 23andMe confirms hackers stole ancestry data on 6.9 million users. TechCrunch. Published December 4, 2023. https://techcrunch.com/2023/12/04/23andme-confirms-hackers-stole-ancestry-data-on-6-9-million-users/

326. Grieg J. 23andMe pledges $30 million to the 6.4 million people affected by data breach. Therecord.media. Published 2023. https://therecord.media/dna-pledges-millions-to-data-breach

327. Imran Rahman-Jones. Genetic testing firm 23andMe investigated over hack. Bbc.com. Published June 10, 2024. https://www.bbc.com/news/articles/c3gg17pq5y9o

328. Bernstein S, Kunkler A, Contursi M. Somebody Spilled the Genes: 23andMe's Downturn Highlights Insufficient Privacy and Data Security Safeguards for Consumer Genetic Data. EPIC - Electronic Privacy Information Center. Published 2024. https://epic.org/somebody-spilled-the-genes-23andmes-downturn-highlights-insufficient-privacy-and-data-security-safeguards-for-consumer-genetic-data/

329. FTC. FTC Says Genetic Testing Company 1Health Failed to Protect Privacy and Security of DNA Data and Unfairly Changed its Privacy Policy. Federal Trade Commission. Published June 15, 2023. https://www.ftc.gov/news-events/news/press-releases/2023/06/ftc-says-genetic-testing-company-1health-failed-protect-privacy-security-dna-data-unfairly-changed

330. FTC. FTC Finalizes Order with 1Health.io Over Charges it Failed to Protect Privacy and Security of DNA Data and

Unfairly Changed its Privacy Policy. Federal Trade
Commission. Published September 6, 2023.
https://www.ftc.gov/news-events/news/press-
releases/2023/09/ftc-finalizes-order-1healthio-over-charges-
it-failed-protect-privacy-security-dna-data-unfairly

Chapter 7

331. Columbia University Irving Medical Center. Study
Identifies Pitfall for Correcting Mutations in Human
Embryos with CRISPR. Columbia University Irving
Medical Center. Published October 28, 2020.
https://www.cuimc.columbia.edu/news/study-identifies-
pitfall-correcting-mutations-human-embryos-crispr

332. Normile D. Chinese Scientist Who Produced Genetically
Altered Babies Sentenced to 3 Years in Jail. Science.
Published December 30, 2019.
https://www.science.org/content/article/chinese-scientist-
who-produced-genetically-altered-babies-sentenced-3-
years-jail

333. Brant R. He Jiankui defends "world's first gene-edited
babies." *BBC News.* https://www.bbc.com/news/world-
asia-china-46368731. Published November 28, 2018.

334. Kolata G, Wee SL, Belluck P. Chinese Scientist Claims to
Use Crispr to Make First Genetically Edited Babies. *The
New York Times.*
https://www.nytimes.com/2018/11/26/health/gene-editing-
babies-china.html. Published November 26, 2018.

335. Greely HT. CRISPR'd babies: Human Germline Genome
Editing in the "He Jiankui Affair." *Journal of Law and the*

Biosciences. 2019;6(1):111-183.
doi:https://doi.org/10.1093/jlb/lsz010

336.Associated Press. First gene-edited babies reported in China. *YouTube.* Published online November 26, 2018. Accessed May 8, 2020.
https://www.youtube.com/watch?v=C9V3mqswbv0

337.Heeren F, J J. Closing the Door with CRISPR: Genome Editing of CCR5 and CXCR4 as a Potential Curative Solution for HIV. *BioTech.* 2022;11(3):25.
doi:https://doi.org/10.3390/biotech11030025

338.Alonso M, Savulescu J. He Jiankui´s gene-editing Experiment and the non-identity Problem. *Bioethics.* 2021;35(6):563-573.
doi:https://doi.org/10.1111/bioe.12878

339.Wannisa Khamaikawin, Chonticha Saisawang, Boonrat Tassaneetrithep, et al. CRISPR/Cas9 genome editing of CCR5 combined with C46 HIV-1 fusion inhibitor for cellular resistant to R5 and X4 tropic HIV-1. *Scientific reports.* 2024;14(1). doi:https://doi.org/10.1038/s41598-024-61626-x

340.Lopalco L. CCR5: From Natural Resistance to a New Anti-HIV Strategy. *Viruses.* 2010;2(2):574-600.
doi:https://doi.org/10.3390/v2020574

341.Baylis F. To publish or not to publish. *Nature Biotechnology.* 2020;38(3):271-271.
doi:https://doi.org/10.1038/s41587-020-0435-1

342.Billauer BP. Responding to the Comeback of He Jiankui, "The CRISPR Baby Scientist": Lessons from Criminal

Justice Theory - Petrie-Flom Center. Petrie-Flom Center - The blog of the Petrie-Flom Center at Harvard Law School. Published March 8, 2023. https://petrieflom.law.harvard.edu/2023/03/08/he-jiankui-crispr-baby-scientist-comeback/

343. Cohen J. Did CRISPR help—or harm—the first-ever gene-edited babies? Science. Published August 1, 2019. https://www.science.org/content/article/did-crispr-help-or-harm-first-ever-gene-edited-babies

344. Georgiou M. Meet Lulu and Nana, the world's first CRISPR genome-edited babies…. Get Animated Medical. Published September 30, 2020. https://getanimated.uk.com/meet-lulu-and-nana-the-worlds-first-crispr-genome-edited-babies/

345. Regalado A. China's CRISPR babies: Read exclusive excerpts from the unseen original research. MIT Technology Review. Published December 3, 2019. https://www.technologyreview.com/2019/12/03/131752/chinas-crispr-babies-read-exclusive-excerpts-he-jiankui-paper/

346. Dimitri Perrin & Gaetan Burgio, The Conversation. New Details About The Infamous "CRISPR Babies" Experiment Have Just Been Revealed. ScienceAlert. Published 2019. https://www.sciencealert.com/china-s-failed-experiment-proves-we-re-not-ready-for-human-gene-editing

347. Wang L, Wang F, Zhang W. Bioethics in China's Biosecurity Law: forms, effects, and unsettled issues. *Journal of Law and the Biosciences*. 2021;8(1). doi:https://doi.org/10.1093/jlb/lsab019

348. BBC. China jails "gene-edited babies" scientist for three years. *BBC News.* https://www.bbc.com/news/world-asia-china-50944461. Published December 30, 2019.

349. Nicolas Gutierrez C. What's next for the gene-edited children from CRISPR trial in China? New Scientist. Published June 29, 2022. https://www.newscientist.com/article/mg25533930-700-whats-next-for-the-gene-edited-children-from-crispr-trial-in-china/

350. Ruwitch J. His baby gene editing shocked ethicists. Now he's in the lab again. NPR. Published June 8, 2023. https://www.npr.org/2023/06/08/1178695152/china-scientist-he-jiankui-crispr-baby-gene-editing

351. Leslie M. Genetically engineered immune cells fight off deadly virus in mice. www.science.org. Published May 2019. https://www.science.org/content/article/genetically-engineered-immune-cells-fight-deadly-virus-mice

352. Palmgren G. News: C46 Boosts CRISPR-Based HIV Resistance - CRISPR Medicine. CRISPR Medicine. Published 2024. Accessed March 3, 2025. https://crisprmedicinenews.com/news/c46-boosts-crispr-based-hiv-resistance/

353. Orit Wolstein, Boyd MP, Millington M, et al. Preclinical safety and efficacy of an anti–HIV-1 lentiviral vector containing a short hairpin RNA to CCR5 and the C46 fusion inhibitor. *Molecular therapy Methods & clinical development.* 2014;1:11-11. doi:https://doi.org/10.1038/mtm.2013.11

354. Tang X, Jin H, Chen Y, et al. A Membrane-Anchored Short-Peptide Fusion Inhibitor Fully Protects Target Cells from Infections of Human Immunodeficiency Virus Type 1 (HIV-1), HIV-2, and Simian Immunodeficiency Virus. *Journal of Virology.* 2019;93(22). doi:https://doi.org/10.1128/jvi.01177-19

355. Paul WE. The Immune System – Complexity Exemplified. *Mathematical Modelling of Natural Phenomena.* 2012;7(5):4-6. doi:https://doi.org/10.1051/mmnp/20127502

356. Dahmer MK, Cornell T, Quasney MW. Genetic and epigenetic factors in the regulation of the immune response. *Current Opinion in Pediatrics.* 2016;28(3):281-286. doi:https://doi.org/10.1097/mop.0000000000000356

357. Deng Linghui, Simin Y, Zhang Zilong, Yuxiao L, Shi Q, Birong D. The relationship between serum klotho and cognitive performance in a nationally representative sample of US adults. *Frontiers in Aging Neuroscience.* 2023;15. doi:https://doi.org/10.3389/fnagi.2023.1053390

358. Kurtzman L. Better Cognition Seen with Gene Variant Carried by 1 in 5 People. Better Cognition Seen with Gene Variant Carried by 1 in 5 People | UC San Francisco. Published May 8, 2014. Accessed March 3, 2025. https://www.ucsf.edu/news/2014/05/114196/better-cognition-seen-gene-variant-carried-1-5-people

359. jpnd. Better cognition seen with gene variant carried by one in five - JPND Neurodegenerative Disease Research. JPND Neurodegenerative Disease Research. Published May 15, 2014. Accessed March 3, 2025.

https://neurodegenerationresearch.eu/2014/05/better-cognition-seen-with-gene-variant-carried-by-one-in-five/

360. Wu F, Pan J, Chen M, et al. Association of serum klotho with cognitive function among individuals with nonalcoholic fatty liver disease. *Frontiers in Aging Neuroscience*. 2024;16. doi:https://doi.org/10.3389/fnagi.2024.1487182

361. Kurtzman L. Smarts and long life, thanks to this gene. University of California. Published May 8, 2014. Accessed March 3, 2025. https://www.universityofcalifornia.edu/news/smarts-and-long-life-thanks-gene

362. Castner SA, Gupta S, Wang D, et al. Longevity factor klotho enhances cognition in aged nonhuman primates. Published online July 3, 2023. doi:https://doi.org/10.1038/s43587-023-00441-x

363. Dubal Dena B, Yokoyama Jennifer S, Zhu L, et al. Life Extension Factor Klotho Enhances Cognition. *Cell Reports*. 2014;7(4):1065-1076. doi:https://doi.org/10.1016/j.celrep.2014.03.076

364. Müller BW, Hinney A, Scherbaum N, et al. Klotho KL-VS haplotype does not improve cognition in a population-based sample of adults age 55–87 years. *Scientific Reports*. 2021;11(1). doi:https://doi.org/10.1038/s41598-021-93211-x

365. Mengel-From J, Soerensen M, Nygaard M, McGue M, Christensen K, Christiansen L. Genetic Variants in *KLOTHO* Associate With Cognitive Function in the

Oldest Old Group. *The Journals of Gerontology Series A: Biological Sciences and Medical Sciences.* 2015;71(9):1151-1159. doi:https://doi.org/10.1093/gerona/glv163

366. Neitzel J, Franzmeier N, Rubinski A, et al. KL-VS heterozygosity is associated with lower amyloid-dependent tau accumulation and memory impairment in Alzheimer's disease. *Nature Communications.* 2021;12(1):1-12. doi:https://doi.org/10.1038/s41467-021-23755-z

367. UCL. How "obesity gene" triggers weight gain. UCL News. Published July 15, 2013. https://www.ucl.ac.uk/news/2013/jul/how-obesity-gene-triggers-weight-gain

368. Su S, Zhao J, Bremner JD, et al. Serotonin Transporter Gene, Depressive Symptoms and Interleukin-6. *Circulation Cardiovascular genetics.* 2009;2(6):614-620. doi:https://doi.org/10.1161/CIRCGENETICS.109.870386

369. Loos RJF, Yeo GSH. The bigger picture of FTO—the first GWAS-identified obesity gene. *Nature Reviews Endocrinology.* 2013;10(1):51-61. doi:https://doi.org/10.1038/nrendo.2013.227

370. Lan N, Lu Y, Zhang Y, et al. FTO – A Common Genetic Basis for Obesity and Cancer. *Frontiers in Genetics.* 2020;11. doi:https://doi.org/10.3389/fgene.2020.559138

371. Huang C, Chen W, Wang X. Studies on the fat mass and obesity-associated (FTO) gene and its impact on obesity-associated diseases. *Genes & Diseases.* 2022;10(6). doi:https://doi.org/10.1016/j.gendis.2022.04.014

372. Karra E, O'Daly OG, Choudhury AI, et al. A link between FTO, ghrelin, and impaired brain food-cue responsivity. *Journal of Clinical Investigation.* 2013;123(8):3539-3551. doi:https://doi.org/10.1172/jci44403

373. Moldovan R, Pintea S, Austin J. The Efficacy of Genetic Counseling for Psychiatric Disorders: a Meta-Analysis. *Journal of Genetic Counseling.* 2017;26(6):1341-1347. doi:https://doi.org/10.1007/s10897-017-0113-8

374. López-Echeverri YP, Cardona-Londoño KJ, Garcia-Aguirre JF, Mary Orrego Cardozo. Effects of serotonin transporter and receptor polymorphisms on depression. *Revista Colombiana De Psiquiatría (english Edition).* 2023;52(2):130-138. doi:https://doi.org/10.1016/j.rcpeng.2021.07.003

375. Virolainen SJ, VonHandorf A, Viel KCMF, Weirauch MT, Kottyan LC. Gene–environment interactions and their impact on human health. *Genes & Immunity.* 2022;24(1). doi:https://doi.org/10.1038/s41435-022-00192-6

376. Hutter C. Gene Environment Interaction. Genome.gov. Published 2024. https://www.genome.gov/genetics-glossary/Gene-Environment-Interaction

377. Dunn A, O'Connell KM, Kaczorowski CC. Gene-by-environment interactions in Alzheimer's disease and Parkinson's disease. *Neuroscience & Biobehavioral Reviews.* 2019;103:73-80. doi:https://doi.org/10.1016/j.neubiorev.2019.06.018

378. Raghavan S, Jablonski K, Delahanty LM, et al. Interaction of diabetes genetic risk and successful lifestyle modification in the Diabetes Prevention Programme. *Diabetes, Obesity and Metabolism.* 2021;23(4). doi:https://doi.org/10.1111/dom.14309

Chapter 8

379. R. Constance Wiener. Newborn genetic testing in the United States and access to needed specialist care, National Survey of Children's Health, 2020: A cross-sectional study. *PLOS ONE.* 2022;17(12):e0279352-e0279352. doi:https://doi.org/10.1371/journal.pone.0279352

380. HRSA. Recommended Uniform Screening Panel | HRSA. www.hrsa.gov. https://www.hrsa.gov/advisory-committees/heritable-disorders/rusp

381. HRSA. Recommended Uniform Screening Panel | Newborn Screening. newbornscreening.hrsa.gov. https://newbornscreening.hrsa.gov/about-newborn-screening/recommended-uniform-screening-panel

382. HHS. Recommended Uniform Screening Panel | Guidance Portal. www.hhs.gov. https://www.hhs.gov/guidance/document/recommended-uniform-screening-panel

383. Singh S, Jelili Ojodu, Kemper AR, Wendy, Grosse SD. Implementation of Newborn Screening for Conditions in the United States First Recommended during 2010–2018. *International journal of neonatal screening.* 2023;9(2):20-20. doi:https://doi.org/10.3390/ijns9020020

384. APHL. APHL. https://www.aphl.org/Pages/default.aspx

385. Chapter 11: Challenges in and Principles for Conducting Systematic Reviews of Genetic Tests Used as Predictive Indicators | Effective Health Care (EHC) Program. effectivehealthcare.ahrq.gov. https://effectivehealthcare.ahrq.gov/products/methods-guidance-tests-genetic/methods

386. Donohue KE, Gooch C, Katz A, Wakelee J, Slavotinek A, Korf BR. Pitfalls and challenges in genetic test interpretation: An exploration of genetic professionals experience with interpretation of results. *Clinical Genetics*. 2021;99(5):638-649. doi:https://doi.org/10.1111/cge.13917

387. Morales A, Hershberger RE. Variants of Uncertain Significance. *Circulation: Genomic and Precision Medicine*. 2018;11(6). doi:https://doi.org/10.1161/circgen.118.002169

388. ACOG. Ethical Issues in Genetic Testing. www.acog.org. Published June 2020. https://www.acog.org/clinical/clinical-guidance/committee-opinion/articles/2008/06/ethical-issues-in-genetic-testing

389. Hauser D, Obeng AO, Fei K, Ramos MA, Horowitz CR. Views Of Primary Care Providers On Testing Patients For Genetic Risks For Common Chronic Diseases. *Health Affairs*. 2018;37(5):793-800. doi:https://doi.org/10.1377/hlthaff.2017.1548

390. Every baby deserves access to genetic screening. *Nature Medicine*. 2024;30(8):2095-2096. doi:https://doi.org/10.1038/s41591-024-03227-9

391. Raspa M, Moultrie R, Toth D, Haque SN. Barriers and Facilitators to Genetic Service Delivery Models: Scoping Review. *Interactive Journal of Medical Research.* 2021;10(1):e23523. doi:https://doi.org/10.2196/23523

392. Alliance G, Health D of CD of. *Newborn Screening.* Genetic Alliance; 2010. https://www.ncbi.nlm.nih.gov/books/NBK132148/

393. Medline Plus. Amniocentesis (amniotic fluid test): MedlinePlus Medical Test. medlineplus.gov. Published 2024. https://medlineplus.gov/lab-tests/amniocentesis-amniotic-fluid-test/

394. CDC. Chorionic Villus Sampling and Amniocentesis: Recommendations for Prenatal Counseling . CDC. Published 2019. https://www.cdc.gov/mmwr/preview/mmwrhtml/00038393.htm

395. Cleveland Clinic. Chorionic Villus Sampling (CVS): What It Is, Benefits & Risks. Cleveland Clinic. Published June 27, 2021. https://my.clevelandclinic.org/health/diagnostics/4028-chorionic-villus-sampling-for-prenatal-diagnosis

396. Zheng Y, Li J, Zhang J, Yang H. The accuracy and feasibility of noninvasive prenatal testing in a consecutive series of 20,626 pregnancies with different clinical characteristics. *Journal of Clinical Laboratory Analysis.* 2022;36(10). doi:https://doi.org/10.1002/jcla.24660

397. Medline Plus. What is noninvasive prenatal testing (NIPT) and what disorders can it screen for?: MedlinePlus

Genetics. medlineplus.gov. Published 2021.
https://medlineplus.gov/genetics/understanding/testing/nipt
/

398. Siva Shantini Jayashankar, Muhammad Luqman
Nasaruddin, Muhammad Faiz Hassan, et al. Non-Invasive
Prenatal Testing (NIPT): Reliability, Challenges, and
Future Directions. *Diagnostics*. 2023;13(15):2570-2570.
doi:https://doi.org/10.3390/diagnostics13152570

399. The American College of Obstetricians and Gynecologists.
The American College of Obstetricians and Gynecologists
- ACOG. Acog.org. Published 2020. https://www.acog.org/

400. ACOG. Screening for Fetal Chromosomal Abnormalities.
Obstetrics & Gynecology. 2020;136(4):e48-e69.
doi:https://doi.org/10.1097/aog.0000000000004084

401. Andrews LB. Social, Legal, and Ethical Implications of
Genetic Testing. Nih.gov. Published 1994.
https://www.ncbi.nlm.nih.gov/books/NBK236044/

402. Genomics England. Newborn Genomes Programme.
Genomics England. Published 2024.
https://www.genomicsengland.co.uk/initiatives/newborns

403. Schaibley VM, Ramos IN, Woosley RL, Curry S, Hays S,
Ramos KS. Limited Genomics Training Among Physicians
Remains a Barrier to Genomics-Based Implementation of
Precision Medicine. *Frontiers in Medicine*. 2022;9.
doi:https://doi.org/10.3389/fmed.2022.757212

404. National Human Genome Research Institute (NHGRI).
Provider Genomics Education Resources. Genome.gov.

https://www.genome.gov/For-Health-Professionals/Provider-Genomics-Education-Resources

405. Sparks TN, Caughey AB. How should costs and cost-effectiveness be considered in prenatal genetic testing? *Seminars in Perinatology*. 2018;42(5):275-282. doi:https://doi.org/10.1053/j.semperi.2018.07.003

406. Guinan S. Costs of Common Prenatal Tests. ValuePenguin. https://www.valuepenguin.com/costs-common-prenatal-tests

407. University of Utah. What is Newborn Genetic Screening? learn.genetics.utah.edu. https://learn.genetics.utah.edu/content/disorders/screening/

408. Oh B. Direct-to-consumer genetic testing: advantages and pitfalls. *Genomics & Informatics*. 2019;17(3):e33. doi:https://doi.org/10.5808/gi.2019.17.3.e33

409. Ayala-Lopez N, Nichols JH. Benefits and Risks of Direct-to-Consumer Testing. *Archives of Pathology & Laboratory Medicine*. 2020;144(10):1193-1198. doi:https://doi.org/10.5858/arpa.2020-0078-ra

410. Nitkin K. Five Things to Know about Direct-to-Consumer Genetic Tests. www.hopkinsmedicine.org. Published March 20, 2018. https://www.hopkinsmedicine.org/news/articles/2018/03/five-things-to-know-about-direct-to-consumer-genetic-tests

411. Cornel MC, van der Meij KRM, van El CG, Rigter T, Henneman L. Genetic Screening—Emerging Issues. *Genes*. 2024;15(5):581. doi:https://doi.org/10.3390/genes15050581

412. National Cancer Institute. Genetic Testing for Hereditary Cancer Syndromes. National Cancer Institute. Published April 18, 2024. https://www.cancer.gov/about-cancer/causes-prevention/genetics/genetic-testing-fact-sheet

413. Franceschini N, Frick A, Kopp JB. Genetic Testing in Clinical Settings. *American Journal of Kidney Diseases.* 2018;72(4):569-581. doi:https://doi.org/10.1053/j.ajkd.2018.02.351

414. Cleveland Clinic. Genetic Counseling. Cleveland Clinic. https://my.clevelandclinic.org/health/articles/23086-genetic-counseling

415. National Human Genome Research Institute. Regulation of Genetic Tests. Genome.gov. Published February 2, 2022. https://www.genome.gov/about-genomics/policy-issues/Regulation-of-Genetic-Tests

416. Yohe S, Thyagarajan B. Review of Clinical Next-Generation Sequencing. *Archives of Pathology & Laboratory Medicine.* 2017;141(11):1544-1557. doi:https://doi.org/10.5858/arpa.2016-0501-ra

417. Satam H, Joshi K, Mangrolia U, et al. Next-Generation Sequencing Technology: Current Trends and Advancements. *Biology.* 2023;12(7):997. doi:https://doi.org/10.3390/biology12070997

418. Churko JM, Mantalas GL, Snyder MP, Wu JC. Overview of High Throughput Sequencing Technologies to Elucidate Molecular Pathways in Cardiovascular Diseases. *Circulation Research.* 2013;112(12):1613-1623. doi:https://doi.org/10.1161/circresaha.113.300939

419. Popova L, Carabetta VJ. The use of next-generation sequencing in personalized medicine. *ArXiv.* Published online March 6, 2024:arXiv:2403.03688v1. https://pmc.ncbi.nlm.nih.gov/articles/PMC10942477/

420. Genomics FL, Higgs M. The Latest Developments in Sequencing Technologies. Front Line Genomics. Published February 6, 2024. https://frontlinegenomics.com/the-latest-developments-in-sequencing-technologies/

421. Slatko BE, Gardner AF, Ausubel FM. Overview of Next-Generation Sequencing Technologies. *Current Protocols in Molecular Biology.* 2018;122(1):e59. doi:https://doi.org/10.1002/cpmb.59

422. 3billion, Inc. 2024 Genome Sequencing Cost Reduction: Advances in AI, CRISPR. 3billion.io. Published 2024. https://3billion.io/blog/whole-genome-sequencing-costs-2024-new-prices-and-future-projections

423. Complete Genomics Incorporated. Next-Generation Sequencing Costs: The Sub $100 Genome. Complete Genomics. Published September 17, 2024. https://www.completegenomics.com/next-generation-sequencing-costs/

424. Weaver J. Cost Comparison of DNA Sequencing Technologies. Base4. Published July 4, 2024. Accessed March 11, 2025. https://www.base4.co.uk/cost-comparison-of-dna-sequencing-technologies/

425. CD Genomics. Sanger Sequencing vs. Next-Generation Sequencing (NGS) - CD Genomics. Cd-genomics.com.

Published 2019. https://www.cd-genomics.com/resource-sanger-sequencing-vs-next-generation-sequencing.html

426. ThermoFisher. What is NGS? - US. www.thermofisher.com. https://www.thermofisher.com/us/en/home/life-science/sequencing/sequencing-learning-center/next-generation-sequencing-information/ngs-basics/what-is-next-generation-sequencing.html

427. Xuchao Z, Zhiyong L, Shengyue W, et al. Application of next-generation sequencing technology to precision medicine in cancer: joint consensus of the Tumor Biomarker Committee of the Chinese Society of Clinical Oncology. *Cancer Biology & Medicine.* 2019;16(1):189. doi:https://doi.org/10.20892/j.issn.2095-3941.2018.0142

428. Mayo Clinic. Clinical Genomics - Overview. Mayo Clinic. Published 2024. https://www.mayoclinic.org/departments-centers/clinical-genomics/sections/overview/ovc-20567367

429. The Johns Hopkins University, The Johns Hopkins Hospital, and Johns Hopkins Health System. Genetics Clinics. Hopkinsmedicine.org. Published 2025. Accessed March 11, 2025. https://www.hopkinsmedicine.org/genetic-medicine/patient-care/genetics-clinics

430. Zalis M, Viana G, Nazareth P, et al. Next-generation sequencing impact on cancer care: applications, challenges, and future directions. *Frontiers in genetics.* 2024;15. doi:https://doi.org/10.3389/fgene.2024.1420190

431. Choon YW, Choon YF, Nasarudin NA, et al. Artificial intelligence and database for NGS-based diagnosis in rare

disease. *Frontiers in Genetics*. 2023;14:1258083. doi:https://doi.org/10.3389/fgene.2023.1258083

432. Park Y, Heider D, Hauschild AC. Integrative Analysis of Next-Generation Sequencing for Next-Generation Cancer Research toward Artificial Intelligence. *Cancers*. 2021;13(13):3148. doi:https://doi.org/10.3390/cancers13133148

433. Sandran NG, Fornarino DL, Corbett MA, et al. Application of multiple mosaic callers improves post-zygotic mutation detection from exome sequencing data. *Genetics in medicine : official journal of the American College of Medical Genetics*. 2024;26(10):101220. doi:https://doi.org/10.1016/j.gim.2024.101220

434. Lu YF ., Goldstein DB, Angrist M, Cavalleri G. Personalized Medicine and Human Genetic Diversity. *Cold Spring Harbor Perspectives in Medicine*. 2014;4(9):a008581-a008581. doi:https://doi.org/10.1101/cshperspect.a008581

435. Baker C, Antonovics J. Evolutionary Determinants of Genetic Variation in Susceptibility to Infectious Diseases in Humans. Knight M, ed. *PLoS ONE*. 2012;7(1):e29089. doi:https://doi.org/10.1371/journal.pone.0029089

436. Shastry BS. Genetic diversity and new therapeutic concepts. *Journal of Human Genetics*. 2005;50(7):321-328. doi:https://doi.org/10.1007/s10038-005-0264-6

437. Trowsdale J, Knight JC. Major Histocompatibility Complex Genomics and Human Disease. *Annual Review*

of Genomics and Human Genetics. 2013;14(1):301-323. doi:https://doi.org/10.1146/annurev-genom-091212-153455

438. Piertney SB, Oliver MK. The evolutionary ecology of the major histocompatibility complex. *Heredity.* 2005;96(1):7-21. doi:https://doi.org/10.1038/sj.hdy.6800724

439. UC Berkeley. Bottlenecks That Reduced Genetic Diversity Were Common Throughout Human History | Research UC Berkeley. Berkeley.edu. Published 2025. Accessed March 11, 2025. https://vcresearch.berkeley.edu/news/bottlenecks-reduced-genetic-diversity-were-common-throughout-human-history

440. Kirkpatrick M, Jarne P. The Effects of a Bottleneck on Inbreeding Depression and the Genetic Load. *The American Naturalist.* 2000;155(2):154-167. doi:https://doi.org/10.1086/303312

441. Hippensteele A. Genetic Diversity in African Populations Can Advance Precision Medicine Globally. Pharmacy Times. Published February 8, 2025. Accessed March 11, 2025. https://www.pharmacytimes.com/view/genetic-diversity-in-african-populations-can-advance-precision-medicine-globally

442. Jorde L. *Genetic Variation and Human Evolution.*; 2003. https://www.ashg.org/wp-content/uploads/2019/09/genetic-variation-essay.pdf

443. Olivier Sibomana. Genetic Diversity Landscape in African Population: A Review of Implications for Personalized and Precision Medicine. *Pharmacogenomics and Personalized*

Medicine. 2024;Volume 17:487-496.
doi:https://doi.org/10.2147/pgpm.s485452

444. Data Harmonization Challenges in Biomedical Research. Elucidata.io. Published 2023. Accessed March 11, 2025. https://www.elucidata.io/blog/quality-at-scale-the-challenges-of-harmonizing-data-across-platforms

445. Pezoulas VC, Fotiadis DI. The pivotal role of data harmonization in revolutionizing global healthcare: a framework and a case study. *Connected Health And Telemedicine.* 2024;3(2). doi:https://doi.org/10.20517/chatmed.2023.37

446. Mc AM, Amber Hartman Scholz, Mathieu Groussin, Staunton C. Benefit-Sharing by Design: A Call to Action for Human Genomics Research. *Annual review of genomics and human genetics.* Published online April 12, 2024. doi:https://doi.org/10.1146/annurev-genom-021623-104241

447. LeBaron S, Crocker R, Rindra Rakotoarivony, et al. Why community consultation matters in genomic research benefit-sharing models. *Genome Research.* Published online January 1, 2024. doi:https://doi.org/10.1101/gr.278308.123

448. Stein V. Genetic research has a white bias, and it may be hurting everyone's health. PBS NewsHour. Published March 21, 2019. https://www.pbs.org/newshour/science/genetic-research-has-a-white-bias-and-it-may-be-hurting-everyones-health

449. Sawyer A. The Effect of Bias in Genomic Studies. BioTechniques. Published September 24, 2018. https://www.biotechniques.com/news/the-effect-of-bias-in-genomic-studies/

450. Peterson RE, Kuchenbaecker K, Walters RK, et al. Genome-wide Association Studies in Ancestrally Diverse Populations: Opportunities, Methods, Pitfalls, and Recommendations. *Cell.* 2019;179(3):589-603. doi:https://doi.org/10.1016/j.cell.2019.08.051

451. Bazeley R. How do we close the diversity gap?- PHG Foundation. PHG Foundation. Published July 11, 2024. https://www.phgfoundation.org/blog/how-do-we-close-the-diversity-gap-in-genomics/

452. Smith LA, Cahill JA, Lee JH, Graim K. Equitable machine learning counteracts ancestral bias in precision medicine. *Nature Communications.* 2025;16(1). doi:https://doi.org/10.1038/s41467-025-57216-8

453. 1000 Genomes | A Deep Catalog of Human Genetic Variation. Internationalgenome.org. Published 2020. https://www.internationalgenome.org/

454. H3Africa | Human Heredity & Health in Africa | Human Genomic Research. H3Africa. https://h3africa.org/

455. The 1000 Genomes Project Consortium. A Global Reference for Human Genetic Variation. *Nature.* 2015;526(7571):68-74. doi:https://doi.org/10.1038/nature15393

456. Devuyst O. The 1000 Genomes Project: Welcome to a New World. *Peritoneal Dialysis International.*

2015;35(7):676-677.
doi:https://doi.org/10.3747/pdi.2015.00261

457. Hanchard Explores Genomics of African Populations. NIH Record. Published August 15, 2024. Accessed March 11, 2025. https://nihrecord.nih.gov/2024/08/16/hanchard-explores-genomics-african-populations

458. H3Africa program comes to an end, leaving an important genomics legacy. Genome.gov. Published 2022. https://www.genome.gov/about-nhgri/Director/genomics-landscape/nov-3-2022-h3africa-program-comes-to-an-end-leaving-an-important-genomics-legacy

459. National Human Genome Research Institute (NHGRI). Researchers Uncover Genetic Variants Linked to Blood Pressure in African-Americans. Genome.gov. Published 2025. Accessed March 11, 2025. https://www.genome.gov/27532579/2009-release-researchers-uncover-genetic-variants-linked-to-blood-pressure-in-africanamericans

Chapter 9

460. Richardson M, Rind D, Beaudoin FL, Pearson SD, Campbell JD. The Fair Price For One-Time Treatments; How Can We Overcome Existing Market Price Distortions? | Health Affairs Forefront. *Health Affairs Forefront.* Published online 2024. doi:https://doi.org/10.1377/forefront.20230117.110613/full/

461. McPhillips D. FDA approves $3.5 million treatment for hemophilia, now the most expensive drug in the world. CNN. Published November 23, 2022.

https://www.cnn.com/2022/11/23/health/hemophilia-drug-hemgenix/index.html

462. Reuters. $2.1m Novartis gene therapy to become world's most expensive drug. the Guardian. Published May 25, 2019. https://www.theguardian.com/science/2019/may/25/21m-novartis-gene-therapy-to-become-worlds-most-expensive-drug

463. Kansteiner F. Bluebird's estimated $2.1M gene therapy prospect Zynteglo gets cost watchdog's backing. Fierce Pharma. Published April 14, 2022. https://www.fiercepharma.com/pharma/bluebird-bios-pricey-gene-therapy-prospect-zynteglo-gets-cost-watchdog-tailwind

464. Khan A, Riaz R, Saad A, Aymar Akilimali. Revolutionary breakthrough: FDA approves VYJUVEK™, the first topical gene therapy for dystrophic epidermolysis bullosa. *Annals of Medicine and Surgery.* Published online October 18, 2023. doi:https://doi.org/10.1097/ms9.0000000000001422

465. Buntz B. With costs up to $4.5M, cell and gene therapies redefine norms. Drug Discovery and Development. Published March 25, 2024. https://www.drugdiscoverytrends.com/how-price-safety-and-efficacy-shape-the-cell-and-gene-therapy-landscape/

466. Wong CH, Li D, Wang N, Gruber J, Lo AW, Conti RM. The Estimated Annual Financial Impact of Gene Therapy in the United States. *Gene Therapy.* 2023;30. doi:https://doi.org/10.1038/s41434-023-00419-9

467. Top four cell and gene therapy challenges facing healthcare systems — and how to address them. Vizientinc.com. Published 2024. https://www.vizientinc.com/insights/articles/2024/top-four-cell-and-gene-therapy-challenges-facing-healthcare-systems-and-how-to-address-them

468. Barry B. Gene Therapy Costs Skyrocket: Payers Turn to Value-Based Contracting. Software Solutions at i3 Verticals. Published March 2024. Accessed April 2, 2025. https://www.i3verticals.com/gene-therapy-costs-skyrocket-payers-turn-to-value-based-contracting/

469. Myshko D. Value-based Outcomes Contracts Can Address High-Cost Gene Therapies. Managed Healthcare Executive. Published February 15, 2023. Accessed April 2, 2025. https://www.managedhealthcareexecutive.com/view/value-based-outcomes-contracts-can-address-high-cost-gene-therapies

470. AveXis Announces Innovative Zolgensma® Gene Therapy Access Programs for US Payers and Families. Novartis. https://www.novartis.com/news/media-releases/avexis-announces-innovative-zolgensma-gene-therapy-access-programs-us-payers-and-families

471. bluebird bio Announces U.S. Commercial Infrastructure to Enable Patient Access to ZYNTEGLO®, the First and Only FDA-Approved Gene Therapy for People with Beta-Thalassemia Who Require Regular Red Blood Cell Transfusions | bluebird bio, Inc. bluebird bio, Inc. Published 2022. https://investor.bluebirdbio.com/news-

releases/news-release-details/bluebird-bio-announces-us-commercial-infrastructure-enable

472. Pagliarulo N. With $2.8M gene therapy, Bluebird sets new bar for US drug pricing. BioPharma Dive. Published August 18, 2022. https://www.biopharmadive.com/news/bluebird-bio-gene-therapy-price-zynteglo-million/629967/

473. Siegle D. 6 Value-based Care Challenges to Overcome - Vim. Vim. Published June 2024. https://getvim.com/blog/value-based-care-challenges/

474. Bartlett W. Strategies to Overcome the Top 7 Value-Based Care Challenges. www.intelichart.com. Published June 6, 2023. https://www.intelichart.com/blog/strategies-overcome-value-based-care-challenges

475. Cell And Gene Therapy Market Size to Hit US$ 132.6 Billion by 2030, Coherent Market Insights. BioSpace. Published November 8, 2024. https://www.biospace.com/press-releases/cell-and-gene-therapy-market-size-to-hit-us-132-6-billion-by-2030-coherent-market-insights

476. Gene Therapy Market Size, Share & Industry Analysis 2026. Allied Market Research. https://www.alliedmarketresearch.com/gene-therapy-market

477. Rosende G. How a National Risk Pool Can Transform Gene & Cell Therapies. ACHP. Published December 6, 2024. Accessed April 2, 2025. https://achp.org/addressing-the-cost-crisis-in-cell-and-gene-therapies/

478. Phares S, Trusheim M, Emond S, Pearson S. *Managing the Challenges of Paying for Gene Therapy: Strategies for Market Action and Policy Reform President and Chief Executive Officer Institute for Clinical and Economic Review.*; 2024. https://icer.org/wp-content/uploads/2024/04/Managing-the-Challenges-of-Paying-for-Gene-Therapy-_-ICER-NEWDIGS-White-Paper-2024_final.pdf

479. Yoo K, Mehta A, Mak J, Bishai D, Chansa C, Patenaude B. COVAX and equitable access to COVID-19 vaccines. *Bulletin of the World Health Organization.* 2022;100(05):315-328. doi:https://doi.org/10.2471/blt.21.287516

480. WHO. COVID-19 vaccinations shift to regular immunization as COVAX draws to a close. www.who.int. Published December 19, 2023. https://www.who.int/news/item/19-12-2023-covid-19-vaccinations-shift-to-regular-immunization-as-covax-draws-to-a-close

481. Das JK, Chee HY, Lakhani S, et al. COVID-19 Vaccines: How Efficient and Equitable Was the Initial Vaccination Process? *Vaccines.* 2022;11(1):11. doi:https://doi.org/10.3390/vaccines11010011

482. FDA's Innovative Approach to Global Gene Therapy Collaboration. Avance Biosciences. Published January 16, 2024. Accessed April 2, 2025. https://www.avancebio.com/fdas-innovative-approach-to-global-gene-therapy-collaboration/

483. Marks P. *Updates on the FDA's Efforts to Accelerate Advances in Cell and Gene Therapy.*; 2025. https://alliancerm.org/wp-content/uploads/2025/01/ARM-Marks-011325.pdf

484. FDA Takes First Step Toward International Regulation of Gene Therapies to Treat Rare Diseases | Insights | Greenberg Traurig LLP. www.gtlaw.com. https://www.gtlaw.com/en/insights/2024/01/fda-takes-first-step-toward-international-regulation-of-gene-therapies-to-treat-rare-diseases

485. Governor Hochul Launches Next Phase of Long Island's Nation-Leading Cell and Gene Therapy Innovation Hub: New York Biogenesis Park. Governor Kathy Hochul. Published 2024. Accessed April 2, 2025. https://www.governor.ny.gov/news/governor-hochul-launches-next-phase-long-islands-nation-leading-cell-and-gene-therapy

486. Industrializing Autologous Cell and Gene Therapy Manufacturing to Bring Quality Products to Patients. BioSpace. Published May 18, 2022. Accessed April 2, 2025. https://www.biospace.com/industrializing-autologous-cell-and-gene-therapy-manufacturing-to-bring-quality-products-to-patients

487. Fresenius and Ori Biotech Announce Collaboration to Advance Modular, Scalable Manufacturing of Cell and Gene Therapies | FSE. Fresenius.com. Published 2024. Accessed April 2, 2025. https://www.fresenius.com/node/6969

488. Ruggles M. Forge Biologics, Labcorp strike deal for gene therapy development and manufacturing. Manufacturing Dive. Published May 11, 2023. Accessed April 2, 2025. https://www.manufacturingdive.com/news/forge-biologics-labcorp-gene-therapy-development-manufacturing-deal/649980/

489. SNS Insider | Strategy and Stats. Snsinsider.com. Published 2024. Accessed April 2, 2025. https://www.snsinsider.com/reports/cell-and-gene-therapy-manufacturing-services-market-1187

490. Business D. Global Cell and Gene Therapy Manufacturing Market to Reach ~USD 10 Billion by 2032 | DelveInsight. GlobeNewswire News Room. Published March 5, 2025. Accessed April 2, 2025. https://www.globenewswire.com/news-release/2025/03/05/3037668/0/en/Global-Cell-and-Gene-Therapy-Manufacturing-Market-to-Reach-USD-10-Billion-by-2032-DelveInsight.html

491. AMP® Bespoke Gene Therapy Consortium (BGTC). FNIH. https://fnih.org/our-programs/accelerating-medicines-partnership-amp/bespoke-gene-therapy-consortium-bgtc/

492. The Foundation for the National Institutes of Health Announces Selection of Eight Rare Diseases for the Bespoke Gene Therapy Consortium Clinical Trial Portfolio | FNIH. FNIH. Published May 16, 2023. Accessed April 2, 2025. https://fnih.org/news/the-foundation-for-the-national-institutes-of-health-announces-

urrough:ursor:

selection-of-eight-rare-diseases-for-the-bespoke-gene-therapy-consortium-clinical-trial-portfolio/

493. Public-Private Alliance Chooses Eight Rare Diseases for Focused Gene Therapy Development. BioSpace. Published June 16, 2023. Accessed April 2, 2025. https://www.biospace.com/public-private-alliance-chooses-8-rare-diseases-for-focused-development

494. The AcCELLerate Forum To Focus On Creating A Sustainable Ecosystem of Cell and Gene Therapy | NMDP. Nmdp.org. Published 2022. Accessed April 2, 2025. https://network.nmdp.org/news-events/newsroom/the-accellerate-forum-to-focus-on-creating-a-sustainable-ecosystem-of-cell-and-gene-therapy

495. Ossandon H, Armijo N, Vargas C, Repetto GM, Manuel Antonio Espinoza. Challenges for gene therapy in the financial sustainability of health systems: a scoping review. *Orphanet Journal of Rare Diseases*. 2024;19(1). doi:https://doi.org/10.1186/s13023-024-03249-z

496. The estimated annual financial impact of gene therapy in the United States | Technology & Policy Research Initiative. sites.bu.edu. https://sites.bu.edu/tpri/2023/12/07/the-estimated-annual-financial-impact-of-gene-therapy-in-the-united-states/

497. Wehrwein P. Cell and Gene Therapy: Becoming More Ordinary. Still Extraordinarily Expensive. *Managed Healthcare Executive*. 2024;34. Accessed April 2, 2025. https://www.managedhealthcareexecutive.com/view/cell-and-gene-therapy-becoming-more-ordinary-still-extraordinarily-expensive

498. Integrated stakeholder views and challenges | Center for Biomedical System Design. Tuftsmedicalcenter.org. Published 2020. Accessed April 2, 2025. https://newdigs.tuftsmedicalcenter.org/payingforcures/integrated-stakeholder-views-and-challenges/#gsc.tab=0

499. McCune JM, Stevenson SC, Doehle BP, Trenor CC, Turner EH, Spector JM. Collaborative science to advance gene therapies in resource-limited parts of the world. *Molecular Therapy.* 2021;29(11):3101-3102. doi:https://doi.org/10.1016/j.ymthe.2021.05.024

500. *Analytical Fact Sheet Sickle Cell Disease: The Silent Killer in Africa Key Messages.*; 2024. https://files.aho.afro.who.int/afahobckpcontainer/production/files/Regional_Factsheet_on_Sickle_Cell_Disease_EN.pdf

501. Cornetta K, Bonamino M, Mahlangu J, Mingozzi F, Rangarajan S, Rao J. Gene therapy access: Global challenges, opportunities, and views from Brazil, South Africa, and India. *Molecular Therapy.* 2022;30(6). doi:https://doi.org/10.1016/j.ymthe.2022.04.002

502. *Accelerating Global Access to Gene Therapies: Case Studies from Low- and Middle-Income Countries.* https://www3.weforum.org/docs/WEF_Accelerating_Global_Access_to_Gene_Therapies_2022.pdf

503. Bridging The Public Knowledge Gap Around Cell And Gene Medicine. Cellandgene.com. Published 2018. https://www.cellandgene.com/doc/bridging-the-public-knowledge-gap-around-cell-and-gene-medicine-0001

504. Williams J. Tackling the trust gap in genomic medicine. EMJ GOLD. Published August 24, 2022. Accessed April 2, 2025. https://www.emjreviews.com/emj-gold/article/tackling-the-trust-gap-in-genomic-medicine/

505. Hawkins DS. Medical exploitation of Black people in America goes far beyond the cells stolen from Henrietta Lacks that produced modern day miracles. The Conversation. Published August 8, 2023. https://theconversation.com/medical-exploitation-of-black-people-in-america-goes-far-beyond-the-cells-stolen-from-henrietta-lacks-that-produced-modern-day-miracles-200220

506. Wikipedia Contributors. Tuskegee Syphilis Study. Wikipedia. Published September 3, 2020. https://en.wikipedia.org/wiki/Tuskegee_Syphilis_Study

507. Minetti E. Ethical Challenges in Medical Research: Henrietta Lacks and the HeLa Cell Line. AWIS. Published January 26, 2024. https://awis.org/resource/ethical-challenges-medical-research-henrietta-lacks-hela-cell-line/

508. DUTCHEN S. Bridging the Trust Gap. Harvard.edu. Published June 2016. Accessed April 2, 2025. https://hms.harvard.edu/news/bridging-trust-gap

509. Jesse Gelsinger. Wikipedia. Published February 23, 2020. https://en.wikipedia.org/wiki/Jesse_Gelsinger

510. Sibbald B. Death but one unintended consequence of gene-therapy trial. *CMAJ: Canadian Medical Association Journal.* 2001;164(11):1612. https://pmc.ncbi.nlm.nih.gov/articles/PMC81135/

511. Rinde M. The Death of Jesse Gelsinger, 20 Years Later. Science History Institute. Published June 4, 2019. https://www.sciencehistory.org/stories/magazine/the-death-of-jesse-gelsinger-20-years-later/

512. American Cancer Society. CAR T-cell Therapy and its side effects. www.cancer.org. Published November 11, 2024. https://www.cancer.org/cancer/managing-cancer/treatment-types/immunotherapy/car-t-cell1.html

513. Risk of secondary cancers after CAR-T cell therapy low, according to large Stanford Medicine study. News Center. Published May 6, 2024. https://med.stanford.edu/news/all-news/2024/06/car-t-secondary-cancer.html

514. Jones C. New Perspectives on the Risk of Secondary Cancers After CAR T-cell Therapy. American Association for Cancer Research (AACR). Published September 16, 2024. https://www.aacr.org/blog/2024/09/16/new-perspectives-on-the-risk-of-secondary-cancers-after-car-t-cell-therapy/

515. Research C for BE and. FDA Investigating Serious Risk of T-cell Malignancy Following BCMA-Directed or CD19-Directed Autologous Chimeric Antigen Receptor (CAR) T cell Immunotherapies. *FDA*. Published online November 28, 2023. https://www.fda.gov/vaccines-blood-biologics/safety-availability-biologics/fda-investigating-serious-risk-t-cell-malignancy-following-bcma-directed-or-cd19-directed-autologous

516. Treating Lymphoma With CAR-T Cell Therapy. med.stanford.edu.

https://med.stanford.edu/cancer/about/news/lymphoma.ht
ml

517. T-cell Malignancies Represent Small Fraction of the
Reported Secondary Cancers following CAR-T in the
FDA's Adverse Event Reporting System - Hematology.org.
www.hematology.org.
https://www.hematology.org/newsroom/press-
releases/2023/t-cell-malignancies-represent-small-fraction-
of-the-reported-secondary-cancers-following-car-t

518. Secondary Cancer Risk Is Low After CAR T Cell
Treatment: Stanford Study. BioSpace. Published June 13,
2024. Accessed April 2, 2025.
https://www.biospace.com/secondary-cancer-risk-is-low-
after-car-t-cell-treatment-stanford-study

519. Horton R, Lucassen A. Consent and Autonomy in the
Genomics Era. *Current Genetic Medicine Reports*.
2019;7(2):85-91. doi:https://doi.org/10.1007/s40142-019-
00164-9

520. Patient Informed Consent - Sangamo. Sangamo. Published
March 25, 2022. Accessed April 2, 2025.
https://www.sangamo.com/bioethics/patient-informed-
consent/

521. Clarke AJ, van El CG. Genomics and justice: mitigating
the potential harms and inequities that arise from the
implementation of genomics in medicine. *Human
Genetics*. 2022;141(5):1099-1107.
doi:https://doi.org/10.1007/s00439-022-02453-w

522. Baum C. Insertional mutagenesis in gene therapy and stem cell biology. *Current Opinion in Hematology.* 2007;14(4):337-342. doi:https://doi.org/10.1097/moh.0b013e3281900f01

523. Liu A. Sarepta reports one death after patient received DMD gene therapy Elevidys. Fierce Pharma. Published March 18, 2025. Accessed April 2, 2025. https://www.fiercepharma.com/pharma/sarepta-reports-1-death-after-dmd-patient-received-gene-therapy-elevidys

524. Gene Therapy for DMD. TREAT-NMD. https://www.treat-nmd.org/resources-and-support/research-overview/dmd/gene-therapy/

525. Fidler B. Duchenne patient dies after receiving Sarepta gene therapy. BioPharma Dive. Published March 18, 2025. Accessed April 2, 2025. https://www.biopharmadive.com/news/sarepta-elevidys-duchenne-gene-therapy-death-liver-failure/742765/

526. Elevidys (delandistrogene moxeparvovec-rokl) FDA Approval History. Drugs.com. Published 2024. https://www.drugs.com/history/elevidys.html

527. Duan D. Lethal immunotoxicity in high-dose systemic AAV therapy. *Molecular Therapy: The Journal of the American Society of Gene Therapy.* 2023;31(11):3123-3126. doi:https://doi.org/10.1016/j.ymthe.2023.10.015

528. Philippidis A. DMD Patient Dies After Treatment with Sarepta Gene Therapy. GEN - Genetic Engineering and Biotechnology News. Published March 18, 2025. Accessed April 2, 2025.

https://www.genengnews.com/topics/genome-editing/dmd-patient-dies-after-treatment-with-sarepta-gene-therapy/

529. Stansfield N. Patient Dies of Acute Liver Failure After Treatment With Sarepta's DMD Gene Therapy Elevidys. CGTlive™. Published March 18, 2025. Accessed April 2, 2025. https://www.cgtlive.com/view/patient-dies-acute-liver-failure-treatment-sarepta-dmd-gene-therapy-elevidys

530. Bryson S. Sarepta reports death of DMD patient given gene therapy, Elevidys. Muscular Dystrophy News. Published March 19, 2025. Accessed April 2, 2025. https://musculardystrophynews.com/news/sarepta-reports-death-dmd-patient-elevidys-gene-therapy/

531. Ronzitti G, Gross DA, Mingozzi F. Human Immune Responses to Adeno-Associated Virus (AAV) Vectors. *Frontiers in Immunology*. 2020;11. doi:https://doi.org/10.3389/fimmu.2020.00670

532. Seed L, Scott A, Peter M, Tadros S, Hill M, Sortica C. Preparing tomorrow's doctors for the genomics era: A nationwide survey of UK medical students. *Future Healthcare Journal*. 2024;11(2):100133-100133. doi:https://doi.org/10.1016/j.fhj.2024.100133

533. Chichka JK. Genetic Cardiomyopathy Awareness Week - DCM Foundation. DCM Foundation. Published June 22, 2023. Accessed April 2, 2025. https://dcmfoundation.org/gcac-goes-global-genetic-cardiomyopathy-awareness-week/

534. Learn the Connection between Genetics and Cardiomyopathy. Genetic Cardiomyopathy Awareness

Consortium. Published March 20, 2025. Accessed April 2, 2025. https://geneticcardiomyopathy.org/

535. Verdonschot JAJ, Hazebroek MR, Krapels IPC, et al. Implications of Genetic Testing in Dilated Cardiomyopathy. *Circulation: Genomic and Precision Medicine.* 2020;13(5):476-487. doi:https://doi.org/10.1161/circgen.120.003031

536. Haga SB, Rosanbalm KD, Boles L, Tindall GM, Livingston TM, O'Daniel JM. Promoting Public Awareness and Engagement in Genome Sciences. *Journal of Genetic Counseling.* 2013;22(4):508-516. doi:https://doi.org/10.1007/s10897-013-9577-3

537. Duyvendak Karakus. The Impact of Patient Advocacy Groups on Clinical Trial Design and Implementation. *Journal of Evolutionary Medicine.* 2024;12(9). doi:https://doi.org/10.4303/JEM/147685

538. *Public Awareness of Direct-To- Consumer Genetic Tests.* https://hints.cancer.gov/docs/Briefs/HINTS_Brief_24.pdf

539. Jobanputra V, Schroeder B, Rehm HL, et al. Advancing access to genome sequencing for rare genetic disorders: recent progress and call to action. *npj Genomic Medicine.* 2024;9(1):1-3. doi:https://doi.org/10.1038/s41525-024-00410-2

540. Your chances of inheriting a disease-causing gene? There's an app for that | Cold Spring Harbor Laboratory. Cold Spring Harbor Laboratory. Published June 13, 2019. Accessed April 2, 2025. https://www.cshl.edu/labdish/your-

chances-of-inheriting-a-disease-causing-gene-theres-an-app-for-that/

541. Genetics Awareness Project. Miami.edu. Published 2025. Accessed April 2, 2025. https://med.miami.edu/centers-and-institutes/hihg/education-and-training/division-of-genomic-outreach/genetics-awareness-project

542. Division of Genomic Outreach. Miami.edu. Published 2025. Accessed April 2, 2025. https://med.miami.edu/centers-and-institutes/hihg/education-and-training/division-of-genomic-outreach

543. Anderson W. ASHG Issues New Guidance Addressing Underrepresentation in Genomics Research Through Community Engagement. ASHG. Published September 2022. Accessed April 2, 2025. https://www.ashg.org/policy/new-guidance-addressing-underrepresentation-in-genomics-research/

544. Frequently Asked Questions. Miami.edu. Published 2025. Accessed April 2, 2025. https://med.miami.edu/centers-and-institutes/hihg/education-and-training/division-of-genomic-outreach/genetics-awareness-project/frequently-asked-questions

545. DCM Foundation. Mended Hearts & DCM Foundation: Empowering Cardiomyopathy Patients and Families. YouTube. Published September 25, 2024. Accessed April 2, 2025. https://www.youtube.com/watch?v=qx9uOYBVFHo

546. Patient Organizations. DCM Foundation.
https://dcmfoundation.org/patient-support-
resources/additional-support/

547. Genentech: Patient Advocacy. www.gene.com.
https://www.gene.com/patients/giving-patients-a-
voice/patient-advocacy

548. Cure Duchenne. CureDuchenne.
https://cureduchenne.org/

549. Parent Project Muscular Dystrophy (PPMD) | Fighting to
End Duchenne. Parent Project Muscular Dystrophy.
https://www.parentprojectmd.org/

550. Jamal L, Schupmann W, Berkman BE. An ethical
framework for genetic counseling in the genomic era.
Journal of Genetic Counseling. 2019;29(5):718-727.
doi:https://doi.org/10.1002/jgc4.1207

551. Sahan K, Lyle K, Carley H, Hallowell N, Parker MJ,
Lucassen AM. Ethical preparedness in genomic medicine:
how NHS clinical scientists navigate ethical issues. *Journal
of Medical Ethics.* Published online February 6, 2024.
doi:https://doi.org/10.1136/jme-2023-109692

552. Schmidt A. 1 Commentary Citation: Schmidt A. Ethical
challenges in genetic research: Navigating Privacy,
Consent, and Equity. *J Res Rep Genet.* 2024;6(5):230.
doi:https://doi.org/10.35841/aarrgs-6.5.230

553. Views on genetic data & ethics. www.ukbiobank.ac.uk.
Published February 16, 2024.
https://www.ukbiobank.ac.uk/explore-your-

participation/stay-involved/uk-biobank-newsletter-homepage-2023-24/views-on-genetic-data-ethics

554. Fight for justice. The University of Newcastle, Australia. Published October 3, 2023. https://www.newcastle.edu.au/hippocampus/story/2023/fight-for-justice

555. Kathleen Folbigg Exonerated | The Australian Greens. The Australian Greens. Published December 14, 2023. https://greens.org.au/nsw/news/media-release/kathleen-folbigg-exonerated

556. Medline Plus. Huntington's disease: MedlinePlus Genetics. medlineplus.gov. Published July 1, 2020. https://medlineplus.gov/genetics/condition/huntingtons-disease/

557. Myers RH. Huntington's disease genetics. *NeuroRX*. 2004;1(2):255-262. doi:https://doi.org/10.1602/neurorx.1.2.255

558. Huntington's Disease: The Pryce Sisters' Story. www.hopkinsmedicine.org. https://www.hopkinsmedicine.org/health/huntingtons-disease-the-pryce-sisters-story

559. Dove ES, Chico V, Fay M, Laurie G, Lucassen AM, Postan E. Familial genetic risks: how can we better navigate patient confidentiality and appropriate risk disclosure to relatives? *Journal of Medical Ethics*. 2019;45(8):504-507. doi:https://doi.org/10.1136/medethics-2018-105229

560. Gordon DR, Koenig BA. "If relatives inherited the gene, they should inherit the data." Bringing the family into the room where bioethics happens. *New Genetics and Society.* Published online December 13, 2021:1-24. doi:https://doi.org/10.1080/14636778.2021.2007065

561. National Human Genome Research Institute. Privacy in Genomics. Genome.gov. Published February 6, 2024. https://www.genome.gov/about-genomics/policy-issues/Privacy

562. Chary S. Genetic Testing: Is There a "Duty to Warn" At-Risk Family Members? - Petrie-Flom Center. Petrie-Flom Center - The blog of the Petrie-Flom Center at Harvard Law School. Published October 11, 2019. https://petrieflom.law.harvard.edu/2019/10/11/genetic-testing-is-there-a-duty-to-warn-at-risk-family-members/

563. What is informed consent?: MedlinePlus Genetics. medlineplus.gov. https://medlineplus.gov/genetics/understanding/testing/informedconsent/

564. Ormond KE, Borensztein MJ, Hallquist MLG, et al. Defining the Critical Components of Informed Consent for Genetic Testing. *Journal of Personalized Medicine.* 2021;11(12):1304. doi:https://doi.org/10.3390/jpm11121304

565. Exploring the Ethics of Genetic Testing: What Does Consent Mean? Diagnostics from Technology Networks. https://www.technologynetworks.com/diagnostics/articles/exploring-the-ethics-of-genetic-testing-what-does-consent-mean-334320

566. Lucassen A, Parker M. Confidentiality and serious harm in genetics – preserving the confidentiality of one patient and preventing harm to relatives. *European Journal of Human Genetics*. 2003;12(2):93-97. doi:https://doi.org/10.1038/sj.ejhg.5201118

567. Genomic Data Sharing: Balancing Privacy and Research Advancements - DrOmics Labs. Dromicslabs.com. Published June 25, 2024. https://dromicslabs.com/genomic-data-sharing-balancing-privacy/

568. NIH Genomic Data Sharing (GDS) Policy and the Genome-Wide Association Studies (GWAS). Human Research Protection Program (HRPP). Published 2015. Accessed April 2, 2025. https://irb.ucsf.edu/nih-genomic-data-sharing-gds-policy-and-genome-wide-association-studies-gwas

569. Genomic Data Sharing | NIH Office of Intramural Research. Nih.gov. Published 2023. https://oir.nih.gov/sourcebook/intramural-program-oversight/intramural-data-sharing/genomic-data-sharing

570. Gymrek M, McGuire AL, Golan D, Halperin E, Erlich Y. Identifying Personal Genomes by Surname Inference. *Science*. 2013;339(6117):321-324. doi:https://doi.org/10.1126/science.1229566

571. Staff R. NIH implements stricter regulations on controlled-access data - The Reporter. UAB Reporter. Published January 16, 2025. Accessed April 2, 2025. https://www.uab.edu/reporter/campus/take-

note/item/10403-nih-implements-stricter-regulations-on-controlled-access-data

572. Vijay Kumar Malesu. News-Medical. News-Medical. Published February 25, 2025. https://www.news-medical.net/health/UK-Biobank-The-Worlde28099s-Largest-Health-Database-Explained.aspx

573. Kudiabor H. "Anonymous" genetic databases vulnerable to privacy leaks. *Naturecom*. Published online October 14, 2024. doi:https://doi.org/10.1038/d41586-024-03236-1

574. 23andMe data leak. Wikipedia. Published February 17, 2024. https://en.wikipedia.org/wiki/23andMe_data_leak

575. Sergiu Gatlan. 23andMe files for bankruptcy, customers advised to delete DNA data. BleepingComputer. Published March 24, 2025. https://www.bleepingcomputer.com/news/security/23andm e-files-for-bankruptcy-customers-advised-to-delete-dna-data/

576. Schwaller F. What does 23andMe bankruptcy mean for genetic data privacy? dw.com. Published March 27, 2025. https://www.dw.com/en/what-does-23andme-bankruptcy-mean-for-genetic-data-privacy/a-72056522

577. Sircar A. 23andMe Bankruptcy: What Happens To Your DNA Data When A Genetic Testing Giant Fails? Forbes. Published March 25, 2025. https://www.forbes.com/sites/anishasircar/2025/03/25/23and mes-bankruptcy-what-happens-to-your-dna-data-when-a-genetic-testing-giant-fails/

578. dreesen stefan. Navigating the fallout: 23andMe's data breach and the ethics of consumer genetic testing. Hospital

News. Published March 26, 2024.
https://hospitalnews.com/navigating-the-fallout-23andmes-data-breach-and-the-ethics-of-consumer-genetic-testing/

579. Kaur A. 23andMe's DNA database is up for sale. Who might want it, and what for? The Washington Post. Published March 25, 2025. https://www.washingtonpost.com/business/2025/03/25/23andme-data-dna-bankruptcy/

580. Nesi C. Calif. AG issues stark warning to 15 million 23andMe users as bankruptcy looms: "Delete your data." New York Post. Published March 23, 2025. Accessed April 2, 2025. https://nypost.com/2025/03/23/us-news/calif-ag-issues-stark-warning-to-15-million-23andme-users/

581. Fowler GA. Delete your DNA from 23andMe right now. The Washington Post. Published March 24, 2025. https://www.washingtonpost.com/technology/2025/03/24/23andme-dna-privacy-delete/

582. FTC Says Genetic Testing Company 1Health Failed to Protect Privacy and Security of DNA Data and Unfairly Changed its Privacy Policy. Federal Trade Commission. Published June 15, 2023. https://www.ftc.gov/news-events/news/press-releases/2023/06/ftc-says-genetic-testing-company-1health-failed-protect-privacy-security-dna-data-unfairly-changed

583. Staff S. FTC charges genetic testing organization for privacy concerns. Securitymagazine.com. Published June 16, 2023. Accessed April 2, 2025. https://www.securitymagazine.com/articles/99508-ftc-charges-genetic-testing-organization-for-privacy-concerns

584. Farris C. Vitagene. Breaches.cloud. Published June 21, 2023. https://www.breaches.cloud/incidents/vitagene/

585. Anastassia Gliadkovskaya. FTC settles first case on privacy, security of genetic information with 1Health.io. Fierce Healthcare. Published September 11, 2023. Accessed April 2, 2025. https://www.fiercehealthcare.com/regulatory/ftc-complaint-against-genetic-testing-company-1healthio-settled

586. Alder S. FTC Fines Genetic Testing Company for Data Privacy and Security Failures. The HIPAA Journal. Published June 20, 2023. Accessed April 2, 2025. https://www.hipaajournal.com/ftc-fines-genetic-testing-company-for-data-privacy-and-security-failures/

587. Brodwin E. A collaboration between Google's secretive life-extension spinoff and popular genetics company Ancestry has quietly ended. Business Insider. https://www.businessinsider.com/google-calico-ancestry-dna-genetics-aging-partnership-ended-2018-7

588. Hendricks-Sturrup RM, Lu CY. Direct-to-Consumer Genetic Testing Data Privacy: Key Concerns and Recommendations Based on Consumer Perspectives. *Journal of Personalized Medicine.* 2019;9(2):25. doi:https://doi.org/10.3390/jpm9020025

589. Popper B. Google's project to "cure death," Calico, announces $1.5 billion research center. The Verge. Published September 3, 2014. Accessed April 2, 2025. https://www.theverge.com/2014/9/3/6102377/google-calico-cure-death-1-5-billion-research-abbvie

590. A Note On 23andMe's New Collaboration with GSK. 23andMe Blog. Published July 25, 2018. https://blog.23andme.com/articles/collaboration-with-gsk

591. Genetic Property Governance | Yale Journal of Law & Technology. Yjolt.org. Published 2025. Accessed April 2, 2025. https://yjolt.org/genetic-property-governance

592. HIPAA Journal. HIPAA Privacy Rule. HIPAA Journal. Published 2024. https://www.hipaajournal.com/hipaa-privacy-rule/

593. Achieving Genetic Data Privacy Through Enforcement of Property Rights | UC Davis Law Review. Ucdavis.edu. Published 2023. https://lawreview.law.ucdavis.edu/archives/57/1/achieving-genetic-data-privacy-through-enforcement-property-rights

594. 2023 Alaska Statutes :: Title 18. Health, Safety, Housing, Human Rights, and Public Defender :: Chapter 13. Genetic Privacy :: Sec. 18.13.010. Genetic testing. Justia Law. Published 2023. Accessed April 2, 2025. https://law.justia.com/codes/alaska/title-18/chapter-13/section-18-13-010/

595. Mitchell C, Ordish J, Johnson E, Brigden T, Hall A. *The GDPR and Genomic Data Executive Summary Authors*. https://www.phgfoundation.org/wp-content/uploads/2023/10/gdpr-and-genomic-data-exec-summary.pdf

596. Shabani M, Borry P. Rules for processing genetic data for research purposes in view of the new EU General Data Protection Regulation. *European Journal of Human*

Genetics. 2017;26(2):149-156.
doi:https://doi.org/10.1038/s41431-017-0045-7

597. About Concert | Precision Health Policy and Payment Accuracy. Concert. Published June 3, 2024. Accessed April 2, 2025. https://www.concert.co/about/

598. Concert. Connecting the Genetic Health Information Network (a whitepaper) - Concert. Concert. Published May 4, 2017. Accessed April 2, 2025. https://www.concert.co/blog/connecting-genetic-health-information-network-whitepaper/

599. BHI. BHI and Concert Genetics Work to Connect Genetic Health Network. Blue Health Intelligence. Published June 5, 2020. Accessed April 2, 2025. https://bluehealthintelligence.com/case-studies/bhi-claims-data-is-helping-concert-genetics-connect-a-much-needed-genetic-health-information-network/

600. Norstad M, Outram S, Brown JEH, et al. The difficulties of broad data sharing in genomic medicine: Empirical evidence from diverse participants in prenatal and pediatric clinical genomics research. *Genetics in medicine : official journal of the American College of Medical Genetics.* 2022;24(2):410-418. doi:https://doi.org/10.1016/j.gim.2021.09.021

601. WHO releases new principles for ethical human genomic data collection and sharing - European Partnership for Personalised Medicine - EP PerMed. European Partnership for Personalised Medicine - EP PerMed. Published November 22, 2024. https://www.eppermed.eu/news-events/news/who-releases-

new-principles-for-ethical-human-genomic-data-collection-and-sharing/

602. World. WHO releases new principles for ethical human genomic data collection and sharing. Who.int. Published November 20, 2024. https://www.who.int/news/item/20-11-2024-who-releases-new-principles-for-ethical-human-genomic-data-collection-and-sharing

603. WHO Launches Guidance on Human Genome Data Collection, Access, Use, and Sharing - World Patients Alliance. World Patients Alliance. Published November 30, 2024. Accessed April 2, 2025. https://www.worldpatientsalliance.org/news/who-launches-guidance-on-human-genome-data-collection-access-use-and-sharing/

604. Agaram Sundaram Vickram, Sivasubaramanian Manikandan, Richard T, S. Vidhya Lakshmi, Chopra H. Targeted Gene Therapy: Promises and Challenges in Disease Management. *Journal of Bio-X Research*. 2024;7. doi:https://doi.org/10.34133/jbioxresearch.0007

605. Dusic EJ, Theoryn T, Wang C, Swisher EM, Bowen DJ. Barriers, interventions, and recommendations: Improving the genetic testing landscape. *Frontiers in Digital Health*. 2022;4. doi:https://doi.org/10.3389/fdgth.2022.961128

606. Suther S, Kiros GE. Barriers to the use of genetic testing: A study of racial and ethnic disparities. *Genetics in Medicine*. 2009;11(9):655-662. doi:https://doi.org/10.1097/gim.0b013e3181ab22aa

607. National Cancer Institute. BRCA mutations: Cancer risk & genetic testing. National Cancer Institute. Published 2024. https://www.cancer.gov/about-cancer/causes-prevention/genetics/brca-fact-sheet

608. Mainor CB, Isaacs C. Risk Management for BRCA1/BRCA2 Mutation Carriers Without and With Breast Cancer. *Current Breast Cancer Reports*. Published online February 17, 2020. doi:https://doi.org/10.1007/s12609-019-00350-2

609. Parkview Health joins Helix Research Network to advance genomic research and precision medicine | Parkview Health. Parkview. Published 2025. Accessed April 2, 2025. https://www.parkview.com/news/results/01152025-parkview-health-joins-helix-research-network-to-advance

610. Sandler S, Alfino L, Saleem M. The importance of preventative medicine in conjunction with modern day genetic studies. *Genes & Diseases*. 2018;5(2):107-111. doi:https://doi.org/10.1016/j.gendis.2018.04.002

611. Caudle KE, Keeling NJ, Klein TE, Whirl-Carrillo M, Pratt VM, Hoffman JM. Standardization can accelerate the adoption of pharmacogenomics: current status and the path forward. *Pharmacogenomics*. 2018;19(10):847-860. doi:https://doi.org/10.2217/pgs-2018-0028

612. National Academies of Sciences E, Division H and M, Policy B on HS, Health R on G and P. *Introduction and Overview*. National Academies Press (US); 2018. https://www.ncbi.nlm.nih.gov/books/NBK538452/

613. Khoury MJ, Bowen S, Dotson WD, et al. Health equity in the implementation of genomics and precision medicine: A public health imperative. *Genetics in Medicine.* 2022;24(8). doi:https://doi.org/10.1016/j.gim.2022.04.009

614. Community. Secondary Genetic Findings: Do You Want to Know? - Mayo Clinic News Network. Mayo Clinic News Network. Published July 20, 2015. Accessed April 2, 2025. https://newsnetwork.mayoclinic.org/discussion/secondary-genetic-findings-do-you-want-to-know/

615. Beshir L. A Framework to Ethically Approach Incidental Findings in Genetic Research. *EJIFCC.* 2020;31(4):302. https://pmc.ncbi.nlm.nih.gov/articles/PMC7745305/

616. Lorenzo D, Esquerda M, Bofarull M, et al. The reuse of genetic information in research and informed consent. *European Journal of Human Genetics.* Published online September 13, 2023:1-5. doi:https://doi.org/10.1038/s41431-023-01457-y

617. The DNA of Genetic Privacy Legislation: Montana, Tennessee, Texas, and Virginia Enter 2024 with New Genetic Privacy Laws Incorporating FPF's Best Practices - Future of Privacy Forum. https://fpf.org/. https://fpf.org/blog/the-dna-of-genetic-privacy-legislation-montana-tennessee-texas-and-virginia-enter-2024-with-new-genetic-privacy-laws-incorporating-fpfs-best-practices/

618. Murthy VS. Exploring Strategies to Increase Genomic Literacy and Integrate Genomic Medicine Education into Graduate Medical Education Programs: A Multi-Case Qualitative Study. Health Sciences Research Commons.

Published 2024. Accessed April 2, 2025.
https://hsrc.himmelfarb.gwu.edu/smhs_crl_dissertations/31/

619. Sirisena ND, Dissanayake VHW. Strategies for Genomic Medicine Education in Low- and Middle-Income Countries. *Frontiers in Genetics.* 2019;10. doi:https://doi.org/10.3389/fgene.2019.00944

620. Training Modules in Genomic Medicine for Healthcare Professionals. Genome.gov. Published 2021. https://www.genome.gov/careers-training/Modules-in-Genomic-Medicine-for-Healthcare-Professionals

621. Schaibley VM, Ramos IN, Woosley RL, Curry S, Hays S, Ramos KS. Limited Genomics Training Among Physicians Remains a Barrier to Genomics-Based Implementation of Precision Medicine. *Frontiers in Medicine.* 2022;9. doi:https://doi.org/10.3389/fmed.2022.757212

622. Karam PE, Hamad L, Elsherif M, et al. Genetic literacy among primary care physicians in a resource-constrained setting. *BMC medical education.* 2024;24(1). doi:https://doi.org/10.1186/s12909-024-05110-0

623. Medical Genetics Awareness Week. Acmg.net. Published 2019. Accessed April 2, 2025. https://www.acmg.net/ACMG/Advocacy/Medical_Genetics _Awareness_Week/MedicalGeneticsAwareness.aspx?hkey= c3c6047a-d7f9-4663-b47a-992af6de2561

624. Helix, Sanford Health Partner on 100K Population Genomics Health Initiative in Upper Midwest. GenomeWeb. Published December 14, 2023. Accessed April 2, 2025.

https://www.genomeweb.com/sequencing/helix-sanford-health-partner-100k-population-genomics-health-initiative-upper-midwest

625. Raths D. Three Health Systems Join Helix Research Network. Hcinnovationgroup.com. Published January 15, 2025. Accessed April 2, 2025. https://www.hcinnovationgroup.com/clinical-it/genomics-precision-medicine/news/55261164/three-health-systems-join-helix-research-network

626. Hewett M. PharmGKB: the Pharmacogenetics Knowledge Base. *Nucleic Acids Research*. 2002;30(1):163-165. doi:https://doi.org/10.1093/nar/30.1.163

627. Landrum MJ, Kattman BL. ClinVar at five years: Delivering on the promise. *Human Mutation*. 2018;39(11):1623-1630. doi:https://doi.org/10.1002/humu.23641

628. Labcorp. Integrating genetic testing into EHR systems | Invitae | Health decoded. Medium. Published April 23, 2024. Accessed April 2, 2025. https://blog.invitae.com/how-integrating-genetic-testing-into-electronic-health-record-ehr-systems-can-address-challenges-6d77a6f95ae4

629. Hicks JK, Dunnenberger HM, Gumpper KF, Haidar CE, Hoffman JM. Integrating pharmacogenomics into electronic health records with clinical decision support. *American journal of health-system pharmacy : AJHP : official journal of the American Society of Health-System Pharmacists*. 2016;73(23):1967-1976. doi:https://doi.org/10.2146/ajhp160030

630. Electronic Health Record-linked Decision Support for Communicating Genomic Data | Digital Healthcare Research. Ahrq.gov. Published 2014. https://digital.ahrq.gov/ahrq-funded-projects/electronic-health-record-linked-decision-support-communicating-genomic-data

631. Nishimura AA, Shirts BH, Dorschner MO, et al. Development of clinical decision support alerts for pharmacogenomic incidental findings from exome sequencing. *Genetics in Medicine.* 2015;17(11):939-942. doi:https://doi.org/10.1038/gim.2015.5

632. Robinson DM, Fong CT. Genetics in medical school curriculum: A look at the University of Rochester School of Medicine and Dentistry. *Journal of Zhejiang University SCIENCE B.* 2008;9(1):10-15. doi:https://doi.org/10.1631/jzus.B073004

633. GENETIC COUNSELING PROGRAM. GENETIC COUNSELING PROGRAM. Published 2024. https://geneticcounseling.ucsf.edu/

634. Curriculum. GENETIC COUNSELING PROGRAM. Published 2023. Accessed April 2, 2025. https://geneticcounseling.ucsf.edu/curriculum

635. Pharmacogenomics Certificate. Knowledge Connection. Published April 24, 2024. https://elearning.ashp.org/products/11488/pharmacogenomics-certificate

636. CPIC. Cpicpgx.org. Published 2009. https://cpicpgx.org/

637. Relling MV, Klein TE, Gammal RS, Whirl-Carrillo M, Hoffman JM, Caudle KE. The Clinical Pharmacogenetics Implementation Consortium: 10 Years Later. *Clinical Pharmacology & Therapeutics.* Published online September 28, 2019. doi:https://doi.org/10.1002/cpt.1651

638. Keating NL, Stoeckert KA, Regan MM, DiGianni L, Garber JE. Physicians' Experiences With BRCA1/2 Testing in Community Settings. *Journal of Clinical Oncology.* 2008;26(35):5789-5796. doi:https://doi.org/10.1200/jco.2008.17.8053

639. Hajek C, Hutchinson AM, Galbraith LN, et al. Improved provider preparedness through an 8-part genetics and genomic education program. *Genetics in Medicine.* 2022;24(1):214-224. doi:https://doi.org/10.1016/j.gim.2021.08.008

640. Hawkins AK, Hayden MR. A grand challenge: Providing benefits of clinical genetics to those in need. *Genetics in Medicine.* 2011;13(3):197-200. doi:https://doi.org/10.1097/gim.0b013e31820c056e

641. Henderson H. CRISPR clinical trials: a 2024 update. Innovative Genomics Institute (IGI). Published March 13, 2024. https://innovativegenomics.org/news/crispr-clinical-trials-2024/

642. Endpoints Contributor. Fueling More Breakthroughs: Manufacturing Innovation to Expand Gene Therapy's Reach. Endpoints News. Published January 20, 2025. Accessed April 2, 2025. https://endpts.com/sp/fueling-more-breakthroughs-manufacturing-innovation-to-expand-gene-therapys-reach/

643. Williamson K. Challenges and Opportunities in Cell and Gene Therapy Manufacturing. Pharmafocusamerica.com. Published February 10, 2025. Accessed April 2, 2025. https://www.pharmafocusamerica.com/articles/challenges-opportunities-cell-gene-therapy-manufacturing

644. News: Clinical Update: Gene-Editing Trials for Solid Cancers. CRISPR Medicine. https://crisprmedicinenews.com/news/clinical-update-gene-editing-trials-for-solid-cancers/

645. Gene therapy's new hope: A neuron-targeting virus is saving infant lives. www.science.org. https://www.science.org/content/article/gene-therapy-s-new-hope-neuron-targeting-virus-saving-infant-lives

Image References

1. Maddox B. NOVA | Secret of Photo 51 | Before Watson and Crick | PBS. www.pbs.org. Published April 2003. https://www.pbs.org/wgbh/nova/photo51/before.html

2. Iltis H. File:Gregor Mendel oval.jpg - Wikimedia Commons. Wikimedia.org. Published 2022. Accessed April 16, 2025. https://commons.wikimedia.org/wiki/File:Gregor_Mendel_oval.jpg

3. Images from the History of Medicine (IHM). Thomas Hunt Morgan - Digital Collections - National Library of Medicine. Nih.gov. Published 2025. Accessed April 16, 2025. https://collections.nlm.nih.gov/catalog/nlm:nlmuid-101422222-img

4. Sutori. The Timeline of DNA. Sutori.com. Published 2025. Accessed April 16, 2025. https://www.sutori.com/en/item/oswald-avery-colin-macleod-maclyn-mccarty-501d

5. McCarty M. File:James D Watson and Francis Crick.jpg - Wikimedia Commons. Wikimedia.org. Published 2022. Accessed April 16, 2025. https://commons.wikimedia.org/wiki/File:James_D_Watson_and_Francis_Crick.jpg

6. MRC Laboratory of Molecular Biology. File:Rosalind Franklin (retouched).jpg - Wikimedia Commons. Wikimedia.org. Published 2022. Accessed April 16, 2025. https://commons.wikimedia.org/wiki/File:Rosalind_Franklin_(retouched).jpg

7. Photo 51. Wikipedia. Published July 25, 2020. https://en.wikipedia.org/wiki/Photo_51#/media/File:Photo_51_x-ray_diffraction_image.jpg

8. Green E. Double Helix. Genome.gov. Published 2019. https://www.genome.gov/genetics-glossary/Double-Helix

9. Holmes family. Researchgate.net. Published 2024. https://www.researchgate.net/figure/Photograph-taken-by-F-L-Holmes-of-Matt-Meselson-and-Frank-Stahl-in-1996-standing-at_fig3_8122131

10. Ostrander E. Central Dogma. National Human Genome Research Institute. Published September 6, 2022. https://www.genome.gov/genetics-glossary/Central-Dogma

11. Ganguly P. Transcription. Genome.gov. Published 2022. https://www.genome.gov/genetics-glossary/Transcription

12. Ganguly P. Translation. Genome.gov. Published 2022. https://www.genome.gov/genetics-glossary/Translation

13. Ganguly P. Retrovirus. Genome.gov. Published 2019. https://www.genome.gov/genetics-glossary/Retrovirus

14. National Library of Medicine. Marshall W. Nirenberg. Profiles in Science. https://profiles.nlm.nih.gov/spotlight/jj

15. Gilchrist DA. Mutation. National Human Genome research institute. Published 2019. https://www.genome.gov/genetics-glossary/Mutation

16. the Nobel Foundation. File:Frederick Sanger.jpg - Wikimedia Commons. Wikimedia.org. Published 2022. Accessed April 16, 2025.

https://commons.wikimedia.org/wiki/File:Frederick_Sanger
.jpg

17. Adams D. DNA Sequencing. Genome.gov. Published
September 6, 2022. https://www.genome.gov/genetics-
glossary/DNA-Sequencing

18. Gene Therapy. Yolasite.com. Published 2025. Accessed
April 16, 2025. https://gene-therapy.yolasite.com/ashanti-
desilva.php

19. Jesse Gelsinger and Family. Jesse Gelsinger in Memory.
www.jesse-gelsinger.com. http://www.jesse-
gelsinger.com/jesses-intent2.html

20. LouLou Foundation. Trustees - James M. Wilson.
Louloufoundation.org. Published 2015. Accessed April 16,
2025. https://www.louloufoundation.org/james-wilson.html

21. Green E. Gene. National Human Genome Research
Institute. Published 2019.
https://www.genome.gov/genetics-glossary/Gene

22. National Institutes of Health, United States Department of
Health and Human Services. File:Francis Collins official
photo.jpg - Wikimedia Commons. Wikimedia.org.
Published June 30, 2017. Accessed April 17, 2025.
https://commons.wikimedia.org/wiki/File:Francis_Collins_
official_photo.jpg

23. NASA . File:302852main patrinos-hi.jpeg - Wikimedia
Commons. Wikimedia.org. Published January 12, 2009.
Accessed April 17, 2025.
https://commons.wikimedia.org/wiki/File:302852main_patr
inos-hi.jpeg

24. Austin CP. Phenotype. National Human Genome Research Institute. Published 2019. https://www.genome.gov/genetics-glossary/Phenotype

25. Datt A. Challengers and our Lives. Substack.com. Published May 6, 2020. Accessed April 17, 2025. https://unnati.substack.com/p/challengers-and-our-lives

26. Gunter C. Point Mutation. Genome.gov. Published 2019. https://www.genome.gov/genetics-glossary/Point-Mutation

27. Biesecker L. Insertion. Genome.gov. Published 2023. https://www.genome.gov/genetics-glossary/Insertion

28. Ganguly P. Deletion. National Human Genome Research Institute. Published 2020. https://www.genome.gov/genetics-glossary/Deletion

29. National Human Genome Research Institute. Copy Number Variation (CNV). Genome.gov. Published 2024. https://www.genome.gov/genetics-glossary/Copy-Number-Variation-CNV

30. National Press Foundation. Victoria Gray - National Press Foundation. National Press Foundation. Published November 17, 2023. Accessed April 17, 2025. https://nationalpress.org/speaker/victoria-gray/

31. Smith M. CRISPR. Genome.gov. Published 2024. https://www.genome.gov/genetics-glossary/CRISPR

32. Bagde P, Kavli Prize. Kavli Prize Laureate Emmanuelle Charpentier. www.kavliprize.org. https://www.kavliprize.org/bio/emmanuelle-charpentier

33. National Human Genome Research Institute, Venditti C. Vector. Genome.gov. Published 2019. https://www.genome.gov/genetics-glossary/Vector

34. Voss S. Washington DC Photographer Stephen Voss. Washington DC Photographer Stephen Voss. Published October 25, 2009. Accessed April 17, 2025. https://www.stephenvoss.com/blog/corey-haas-gene-therapy

35. United For Medical Research. Jean Bennett: A Gene Therapy to Treat Blindness - United For Medical Research. United For Medical Research. Published February 5, 2020. Accessed April 17, 2025. https://www.unitedformedicalresearch.org/podcast/jean-bennett-a-gene-therapy-to-treat-blindness/

36. Harvard Ophthalmology Communications Office. Eric A. Pierce, MD, PhD. Harvard.edu. Published 2025. Accessed April 17, 2025. https://eye.hms.harvard.edu/ericpierce

37. Emily Whitehead Foundation. Our Journey. Emily Whitehead Foundation. https://emilywhiteheadfoundation.org/our-journey/

38. Liu PP. Oncogene. Genome.gov. Published 2023. https://www.genome.gov/genetics-glossary/Oncogene

39. Duke Neurosurgery. First patient to undergo poliovirus therapy for GBM dies eight years after treatment. Duke Department of Neurosurgery. Published April 6, 2020. https://neurosurgery.duke.edu/news/first-patient-undergo-poliovirus-therapy-gbm-dies-eight-years-after-treatment

40. Annick Desjardins | Duke Department of Neurosurgery. Duke.edu. Published 2024. Accessed April 18, 2025. https://neurosurgery.duke.edu/profile/annick-desjardins

41. Bates S. Nucleic Acids. Genome.gov. Published 2023. https://www.genome.gov/genetics-glossary/Nucleic-Acids

42. Nobel Prize Outreach. The Nobel Prize in Physiology or Medicine 2006. NobelPrize.org. https://www.nobelprize.org/prizes/medicine/2006/summary/

43. Sen S. Ribonucleic Acid (RNA). Genome.gov. Published 2024. https://www.genome.gov/genetics-glossary/Ribonucleic-Acid-RNA

44. National Human Genome Research Institute. Antisense. Genome.gov. Published 2019. https://www.genome.gov/genetics-glossary/antisense

45. Rady Children's Institute for Genomic Medicine. Fitz's Story | RCIGM. RCIGM. Published October 10, 2024. https://radygenomics.org/case-studies/fitzs-story/

46. Mesa J. Deaf Baby Girl Hears for First Time in "Mind-Blowing" Gene Therapy Trial. Newsweek. Published May 9, 2024. Accessed April 18, 2025. https://www.newsweek.com/regeneron-gene-therapy-baby-girl-deaf-opal-sandy-1898883#slideshow/2390744

47. Cambridge University Hospitals. Baby born deaf can hear after breakthrough gene therapy. Cambridge University Hospitals. Published May 2024. https://www.cuh.nhs.uk/news/baby-born-deaf-can-hear-after-breakthrough-gene-therapy/

48. L'hôpital Necker, les enfants bulles et la thérapie génique : épisode 2/5 du podcast Alain Fischer, l'exigence médicale | Radio France. France Culture. Published 2023. Accessed April 18, 2025. https://www.radiofrance.fr/franceculture/podcasts/a-voix-nue/l-hopital-necker-les-enfants-bulles-et-la-therapie-genique-9257609

49. Mass Chan Medical School. Noa's story. UMass Chan Medical School. Published January 28, 2025. https://www.umassmed.edu/news/rarediseasesrealstories/noas-story/

50. Massachusetts General Hospital. Florian Eichler, MD - Department of Neurology. Massachusetts General Hospital. Published 2024. Accessed April 18, 2025. https://www.massgeneral.org/doctors/17851/florian-eichler

51. Philadelphia TCH of. Gene Therapy for Sickle Cell Disease: Marie-Chantal's Story. www.chop.edu. Published November 22, 2023. https://www.chop.edu/stories/gene-therapy-sickle-cell-disease-marie-chantal-s-story

52. Philadelphia TCH of. Alexis A. Thompson, MD, MPH. www.chop.edu. Published December 10, 2021. https://www.chop.edu/doctors/thompson-alexis-a

53. CDC. Little Feet Make Big Footprints in Health. Newborn Screening. Published 2024. https://www.cdc.gov/newborn-screening/featurestory/little-feet-big-footprints.html

54. CDC. Real Stories About Lynch Syndrome. Hereditary Colorectal (Colon) Cancer. Published October 16, 2024.

https://www.cdc.gov/colorectal-cancer-
hereditary/stories/index.html

55. Phillips N. She was convicted of killing her four children.
    Could a gene mutation set her free? Nature.
    2022;611(7935):218-223.
    doi:https://doi.org/10.1038/d41586-022-03577-9

56. The He Lab. File:He Jiankui (cropped).jpg - Wikimedia
    Commons. Wikimedia.org. Published November 25, 2018.
    Accessed April 22, 2025.
    https://commons.wikimedia.org/wiki/File:He_Jiankui_(cro
    pped).jpg

57. Hurle B. Germ Line. Genome.gov.
    https://www.genome.gov/genetics-glossary/germ-line

58. National Human Genome Research Institute.
    Heterozygous. Genome.gov. Published 2019.
    https://www.genome.gov/genetics-glossary/heterozygous

59. University College London. Ucl.ac.uk. Published 2025.
    Accessed April 22, 2025. https://profiles.ucl.ac.uk/6166

60. Sapp JC. X-Linked. Genome.gov.
    https://www.genome.gov/genetics-glossary/X-Linked

61. Greenwood Genetic Center. Meet Nora - Newborn
    screening and treatment is a literal lifesaver! - Greenwood
    Genetic Center. Greenwood Genetic Center. Published
    April 18, 2025. Accessed April 23, 2025.
    https://ggc.org/patient-stories-1/meet-nora

62. Pathogenic Variant. Genome.gov. Published 2025.
    https://www.genome.gov/genetics-glossary/Pathogenic-
    Variant

63. The Johns Hopkins University. Huntington's Disease: The
    Pryce Sisters' Story. www.hopkinsmedicine.org.
    https://www.hopkinsmedicine.org/health/huntingtons-
    disease-the-pryce-sisters-story

www.ingramcontent.com/pod-product-compliance
Lightning Source LLC
Chambersburg PA
CBHW060834280326
41934CB00007B/783